Embodied Ayurveda for Yoga Practitioners,
Increasing the Healing Potential of Yoga
Copyright ©2021 by Faye Berton. All rights reserved.

Paperback ISBN 978-0-9990340-2-6

www.fayeberton.com

Edited by Karin Preus, Katie Charlet & Kevin Coughlin
Book design by Karin Preus/Acorn Design
Photoshop collages by Karin Preus
VPK models Cheryl Ekstrum, Mary Ann Bradley, Liz Liddiard Wozniak
VPK model photographs by Larry Marcus
Faye asana photographs by George Peer

Embodied Ayurveda for Yoga Practitioners

Increasing the Healing Potential of Yoga

Faye Berton

LAUREL PRESS

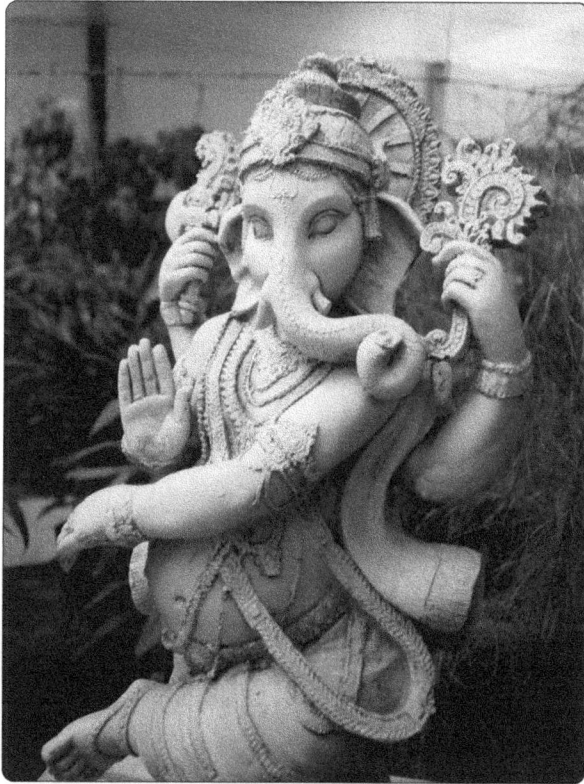

*Dedicated to all people
who use this book
in support of healing themselves
and others.*

Table of Contents

INTRODUCTIONS

YOGA, AYURVEDA & SOMATIC AWARENESS

PART ONE: AYURVEDIC ANATOMY & PHYSIOLOGY

⮑ ELEMENTS

⮑ DOSHAS

"Ayurveda" *is a traditional, holistic medical system from India that emerged from the same philosophical ground as yoga.*

The word Ayurveda is made up of two Sanskrit words: **"ayu"** *meaning life, longevity and* **"veda"** *meaning knowledge or science.*

Thus, Ayurveda is the knowledge or science of creating health, vitality and long life.

Is This Book for You?

As yoga practitioners, we intuitively adapt our practice to how we are feeling.

If we are low in energy we will do a less vigorous practice. A restorative practice is more appealing when we are not feeling well. When we are stressed, we might be attracted to a challenging practice to wash away the tension, or to a gentle practice to soothe our body/mind. All of this is common sense and instinct.

The goal of this book is to help people bring this common sense/instinct into full consciousness and, using Ayurveda, further develop it.

A beginning practitioner can integrate Ayurvedic principles into their learning of yoga. Established practitioners will discover a world of subtle adjustments and focuses that they can use to add freshness, breadth and healing potency to their practice.

Embodying Ayurveda gives yoga practitioners powerful self-care tools and provides yoga teachers with the knowledge of how to tailor practices to the needs of their students.

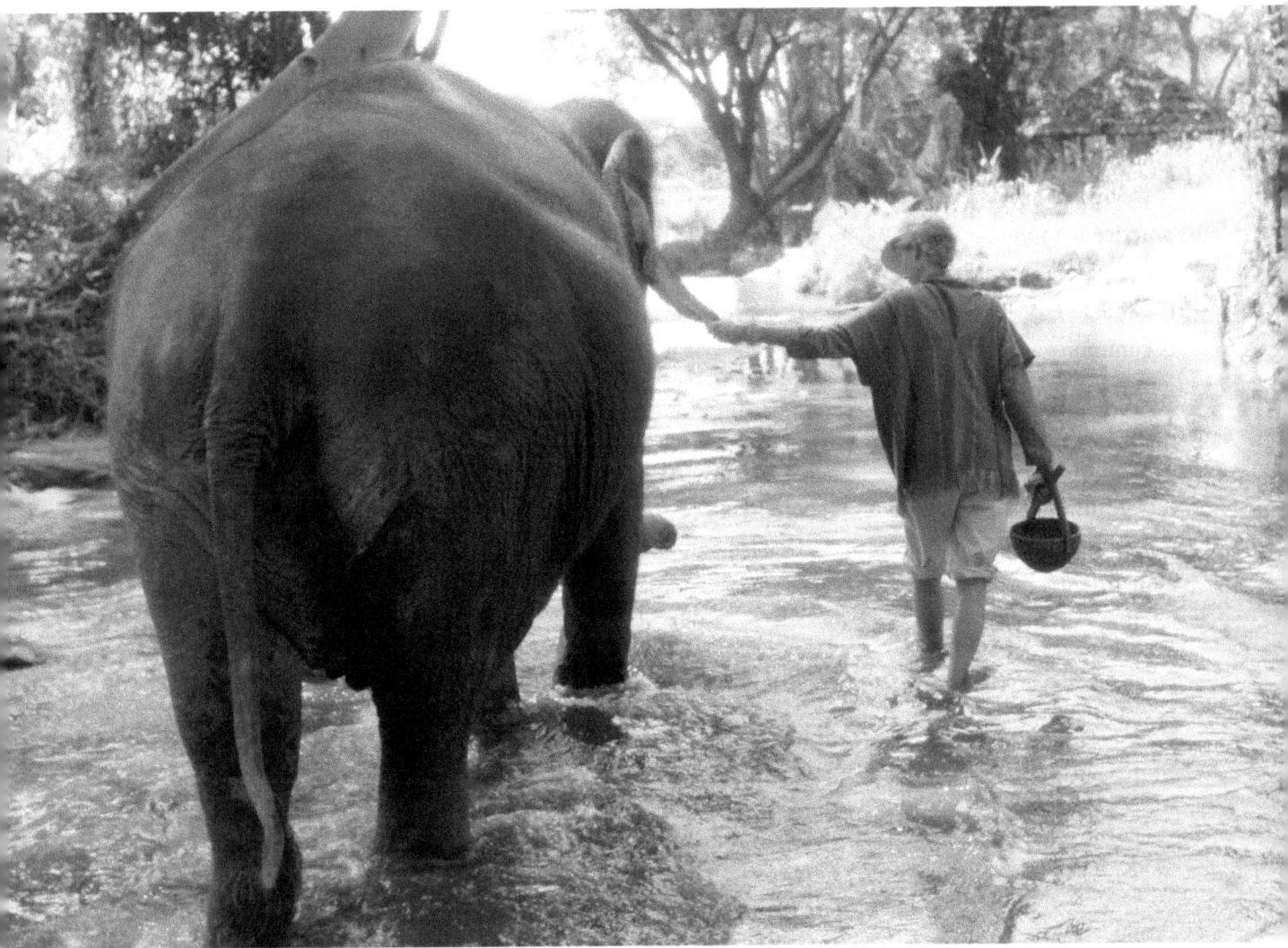

The author in Thailand

The Author's Journey –
Yoga, Ayurveda & Somatic Disciplines

Yoga

I came to yoga through Swami Vivekananda's little orange book on Raja yoga. I was sixteen and I purchased the book through an advertisement in the back of a magazine.

Yoga has been central in my life now for over fifty years, and it has been my livelihood for thirty years. I love the challenge of new and more complex practices and am nourished by the simple and familiar. Yoga philosophy is the world view to which I subscribe.

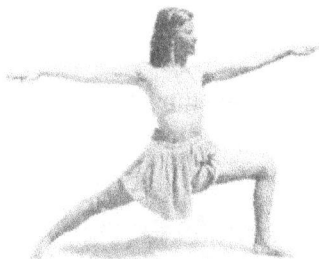

Over the years I have enthusiastically explored many styles of yoga with many different teachers. Years of weekly study with Swami Veda Bharati gave me a solid foundation in traditional yoga philosophy. I gained understanding of working with structural intelligence of the body though trainings with senior Iyengar teachers. Yogi Bhajan gave me experience of the aliveness that is possible when vigorous breathing is coupled with movement.

Injuries and illnesses have been catalysts through which my practice and understanding developed. A basic asana practice was my primary support in getting through two years of chronic fatigue. A knee injury that refused to heal through physical therapy resolved easily in a month of meditative asana work.

Two milestones signaled major shifts in my yogic journey. One was discovering the world of somatic awareness, the other was fulfilling a dream of studying Ayurveda with Dr. Vasant Lad.

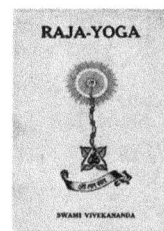

Somantic Awareness

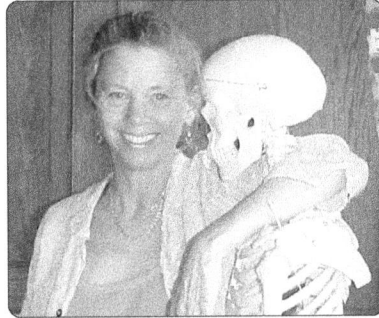

I was introduced to the world of somatic awareness by a demonstration of the Alexander Technique at a yoga center. That experience turned my life in a new direction. The Technique gave me an experience of ease in my body which I then began looking for in my yoga practice. In that process asana became easier, more enjoyable and more effective. My meditation also became deeper and quieter. That was the first step in what became an intensive journey in learning about somatic awareness.

A serious shoulder injury that would not resolve prompted my osteopath to refer me to the Feldenkrais Method. Through the Feldenkrais Method I learned new ways of thinking about the body, breath, movement and yoga. I learned about *learning how to learn* and began understanding how to *think* through my body. I not only resolved my shoulder injury through Feldenkrais, but my yoga practice blossomed exponentially in richness, subtlety and effectiveness.

A deeper exploration of **somatic awareness** appears on page 29.

The Feldenkrais Method is my primary somatic discipline, but I have also had the good fortune to study in some depth with masters of other somatic disciplines, which include: The Alexander Technique with Marjorie Barstow, Continuum Movement with Emilie Conrad, Somatic Awareness with Charlotte Selver, Breathexperience with Elsa Middendorf, Rubenfeld Synergy with Ilana Rubenfeld, and Bones for Life with Ruthy Alon.

I started teaching yoga at the same time I started learning about somatic disciplines and so somatic awareness has been integral to my teaching of yoga from day one.

Ayurveda

I was introduced to Ayurveda through a weekend workshop with Robert Svoboda in the early-80s. I was smitten! At that time there were very few options for learning about Ayurveda. I worked with what was available then but that did not get me very far.

Finally, in 2001, life opened a door for me to go to the Ayurvedic Institute and study with Dr. Lad. During my time at the Institute I had a conversation with David Frawley about my work with somatic awareness and yoga. I knew that somatic awareness was important to me both in my personal development as well as in how I practiced and taught yoga. I felt some slight discomfort, however, because I didn't know how to think about the relationship between somatic awareness and yoga. I also had an inkling of concern that I might be diluting my yoga practice with a *non-yogic* practice.

When I expressed this angst to David, his immediate and clear response surprised me — "in somatic disciplines," he said, "you are cultivating the *subtle body*." It was a wonderful moment for me, both in feeling relieved for having my work affirmed and for the understanding I gained about somatic awareness and its relationship to yoga.

As a giant bonus in this epiphanic moment, I also realized that in studying Ayurveda I was learning *Ayurveda's view of the subtle body*. Ayurveda engages the underlying energies of health and disease, and those energies are the subtle body. My understanding of Ayurveda took an exponential leap.

Ayurveda engages the underlying energies of health and disease, and those energies are the subtle body.

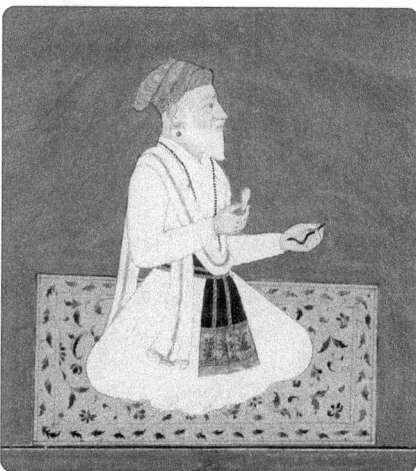

Dhanvantari, the founder of Ayurveda

At this point, yoga, somatic awareness and Ayurveda live in me as a single weave. If I pull on a thread of one of these systems, I am tugging on the others. It is out of this tapestry of yoga, somatic awareness and Ayurveda that the material in this book has emerged.

I hope you find it useful.

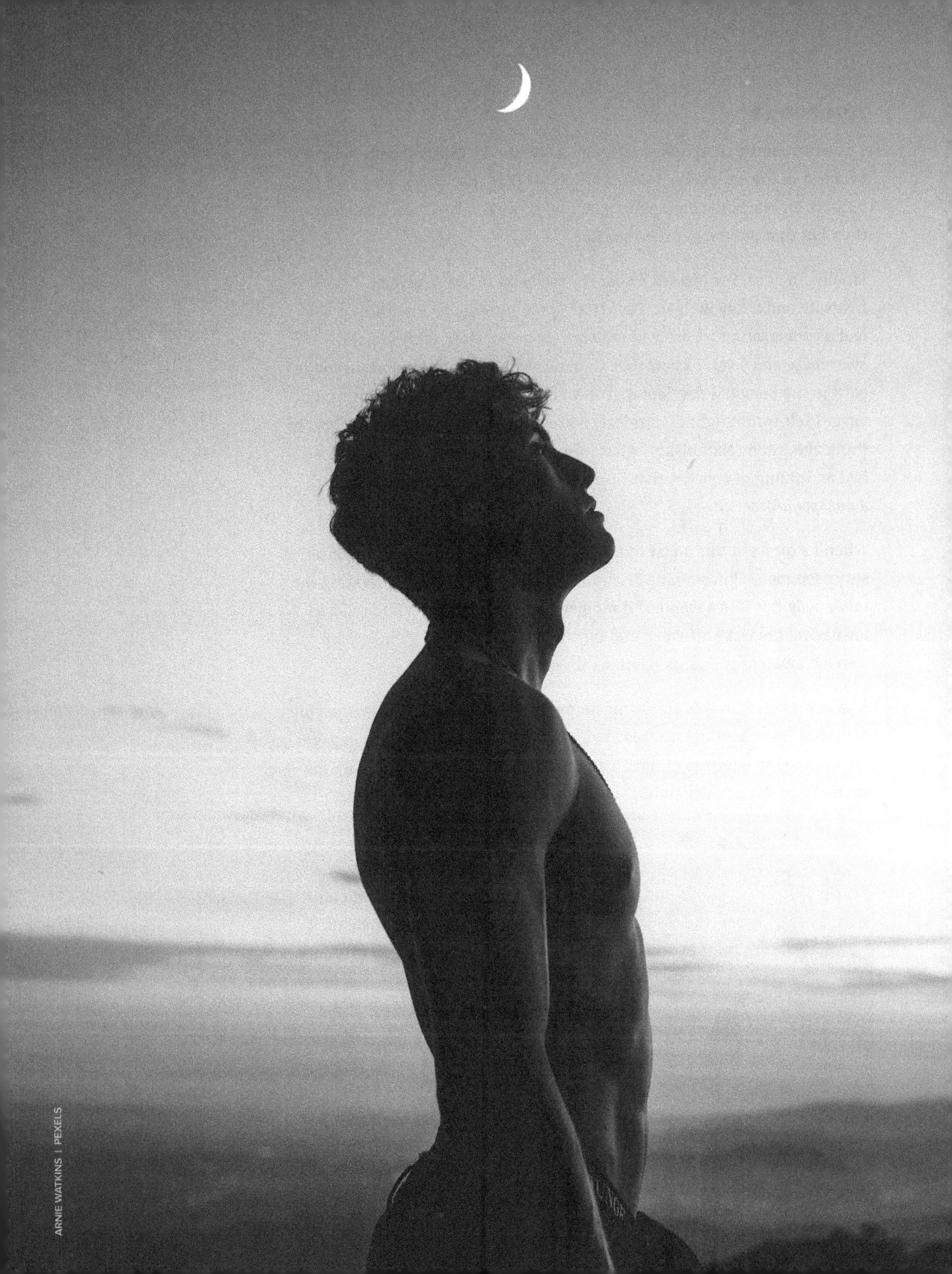

It's All About Awareness

Integrating Ayurveda into the practice of yoga is a matter of learning Ayurvedic principles, exploring these principles as living processes in our own body, and then bringing them into our yoga practice.

The process described in this book uses somatic awareness to explore Ayurvedic principles as an internal experience.

In their unique ways, all three of these — yoga, Ayurveda and somatic disciplines — are about awareness.

Yoga done as exercise is about awareness of the body and breath. Traditionally speaking, the goal of Yoga is awareness of our whole self. Patanjali, author of the *Yoga Sutras*, describes a process by which we first become aware of our relationship to others and to ourselves; then we cultivate awareness of our body and breath; finally, we develop awareness of the different levels of our mind.

Ayurveda is about developing awareness of how we relate to ourselves and our world. Everything we do and everything in our world affects the state of our body/mind, and so affects our experience of life. It is only through self-awareness that we can recognize and make changes in how we relate to ourselves and our world, and it is only with this recognition that we can achieve high-level health and happiness.

The goal of **somatic disciplines** is cultivating somatic awareness. Somatic awareness is being in touch with the felt-sense of being alive. It is about experiencing our bodies as living intelligence that communicates to us through the language of sensation. It is through sensation that we are aware of what is happening inside our skin. Somatic awareness is the same as embodied awareness.

This Book in a Nutshell

The starting point for this book is a brief overview of **Yoga and Ayurveda,** along with a discussion of their natural relationship and their overlapping goals.

Moving on to **Ayurvedic Anatomy and Physiology**, you will learn about three primary principles of Ayurveda. Understanding these principles and cultivating awareness of them as living processes inside yourself is the foundation for bringing Ayurveda into the practice of yoga.

These principles are:

- The **FIVE ELEMENTS**
- The **THREE DOSHAS**
- The **FIVE PRANAS**

The Five Elements, sometimes called the Five Great Elements, are not the elements that we know from the natural world. The Five Great Elements are rather the energies/substances out of which everything in the natural world arises.

The Three Doshas form Ayurveda's signature principle. The Doshas are a way of describing how the Five Elements function in our body, mind and emotions.

Prana is our life-energy, and the Five Pranas are the five major directions in which prana flows in our body. Prana is an expression of the air element.

The last section of the book is devoted to **practices**. This section offers three levels of practice for developing skill in applying Ayurveda to yoga. These levels are:

- ❧ **Practice FOCUSES**
- ❧ **Practice SEEDS**
- ❧ **Practice SEQUENCES**

Practice Focuses are an overview of different ways of using your attention in asana. Working with the Focuses is a means of both cultivating *somatic awareness* and of influencing the effect of a practice. Three types of Focuses are presented:

- ❧ **Physical Focuses**
- ❧ **Energetic/Breath Focuses**
- ❧ **Mental/Emotional Focuses**

Practice Seeds are Ayurvedic principles that can easily be included in your regular yoga practice. You can include one or many Seeds depending on your interests and needs. Practice Seeds allow you to explore Ayurveda and yoga together at a relaxed pace within the comfort of a familiar practice.

Practice Sequences are structured yoga practices that are composed primarily of asanas chosen for their Ayurvedic balancing effect. A few breathing and meditation practices are also included. Practice Focuses and Practice Seeds are integrated into the Sequences in order to increase their Ayurvedic balancing effect.

The asanas in the Sequences are purposefully simple to make it easier to sustain attention on your inner experience.

Making This Book Useful

I am lucky, I had two years to absorb this book. As Faye sent me pages, chapters, thoughts, big pictures — I soaked. Reading it required my full attention, each paragraph. It did not require that I finish more than one paragraph in any prescribed time frame. I took it at a ponderer's pace. That is one way you could choose to encounter this book.

We did a number of things to try to slow the pace — adding engaging photographs, poetry, quotations. Faye says one of the traditional ways yoga was taught was by *osmosis*. Gaze. Spend time. Meditate. Language is necessary but it is only cognitive and thus limiting. Images, on the other hand, can go deeper into the nervous system, further illuminating and supporting our understanding.

We dug and dug for images that would serve as reflections of the words, and then be captivating enough to invite you to pause. And then gaze. Make some tea. Re-read a paragraph. Look out the window. Realize — in that slow, bubbling-up, wonderful way — that there is this whispering, tiny connection between that pain in your elbow and your vata constitution!

This book ended up being a companion rather than something to *accomplish* (being a pitta, the latter is my default). I was able to employ the ideas and practices in the book in a natural progression — learning, one digestible bite at a time, as Feldenkrais recommends. This "relationship" allowed for integration at a deeper and more sustainable level, one that becomes not just a part of my practice, but my dish-washing, my encounters with dear ones, my capacity for self-care, and on and on.

This is a book to be read, one from which to practice and one to use as an insightful resource. There are way-finding devices I employed to keep my own head from blowing up as the book took shape. On each lower-left page you will find what *section* you're in. On the lower right, you'll find the chapter. At the start of Part Two, there is a Table of Practices. I hope this helps you sort *Seeds* from *Sequences*.

As a practitioner, I know the fumbling hilarity of trying to learn something new as I lie on the floor. So the font is on the large side. There are tabs and references (ⓘ), indexes and tables that I hope will serve you like devoted breadcrumbs.

These devices reflect solutions from a designer's perspective but also how I was able to make the material useful to me as a reader and student, each and every day. I wish you the same.

Karin Preus, Designer

A Note on Ayurveda

Ayurveda is a traditional holistic medical system with a comprehensive understanding of how to create high-level health and wellness. It is effective for both preventing and recovering from disease.

Yoga is an important part of Ayurvedic treatment plans, but it is only a part. Someone who is interested in using Ayurveda for addressing a challenging health concern would want to find an Ayurvedic doctor.

Ayurveda treatment plans are holistic. Along with the yoga practices of asana, pranayama and meditation, they include diet, herbs, gems, life-style recommendations and a variety of bodywork practices.

This book is limited to a basic understanding of Ayurvedic principles and how to use these principles to expand the healing potential of yoga.

Significant health benefit can be gained from working with the practices in this book, but addressing a complex health problem requires a complete Ayurvedic treatment plan. See the Appendix, page 231, for reference.

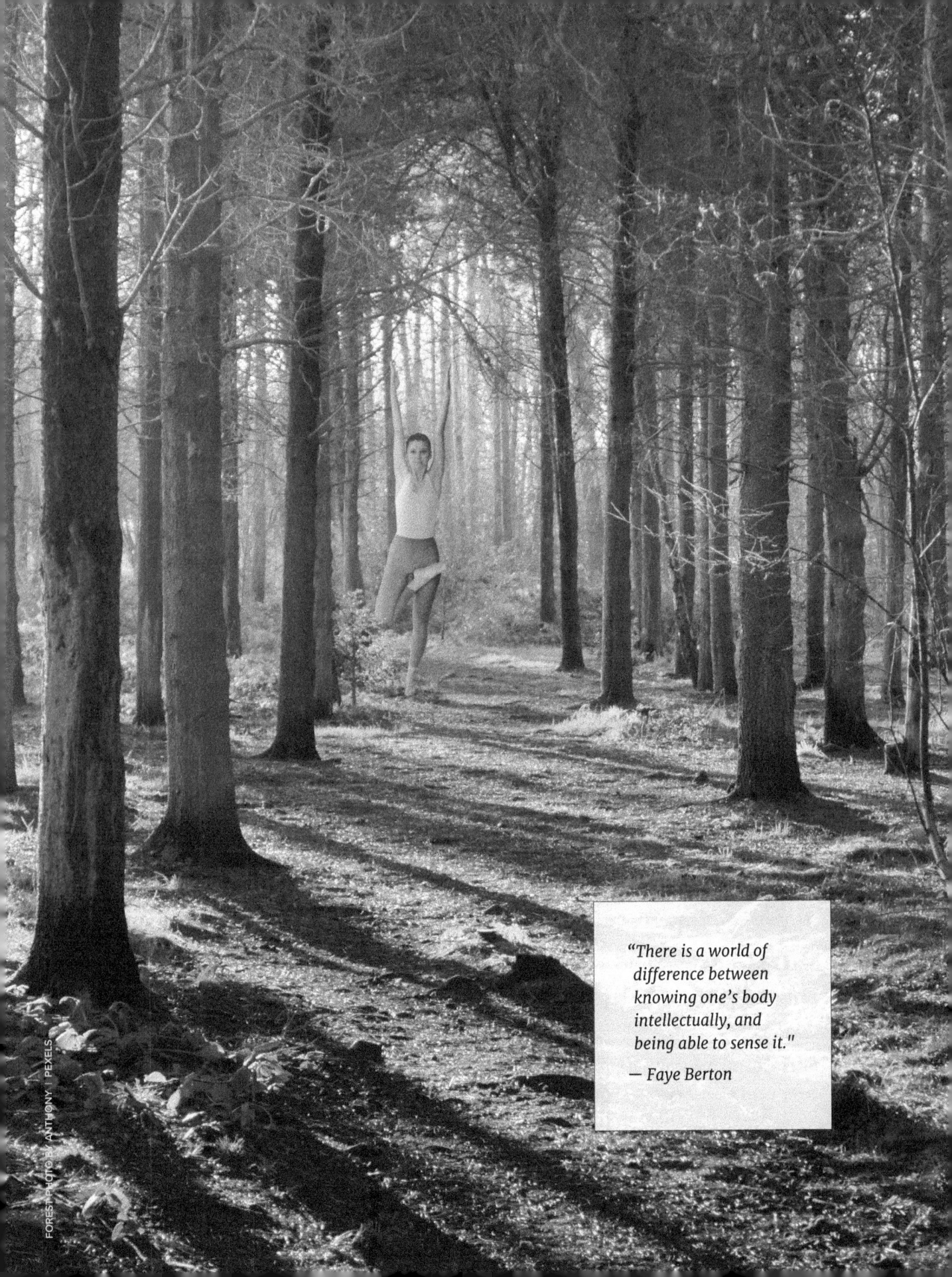

> "There is a world of
> difference between
> knowing one's body
> intellectually, and
> being able to sense it."
>
> — Faye Berton

Yoga & Ayurveda – A Natural Relationship

Just as light refracting through a prism expresses as different colors, so Ayurveda and Yoga are two wisdom traditions that emerged from a single philosophy. This shared philosophy allows for a natural ease of communication between them.

Enhancing Yoga with Ayurveda

The cultivation of health, wholeness and joy are goals shared by both yoga and Ayurveda. Health creates vitality, experiencing our wholeness creates contentment and joy gives us radiance. Health, wholeness and joy are at the heart of a fulfilled life. With them we need little else, without them our needs feel endless.

Health, wholeness and joy are our birthright, but they are not automatic. We must decide we want them, then choose a reliable source of guidance to help us access them. The former is up to us, Yoga and Ayurveda can provide the latter.

The Ayurvedic and Yogic approaches to health, wholeness and joy are different but overlapping. Ayurveda is a medical system that focuses on creating health, happiness and longevity. Yoga is a discipline that provides us with practices for refining our body, breath and mind. Each of these systems alone is effective in helping us create a fulfilled life, but together they are even more effective. Each system benefits by including some of the practices of the other.

Ayurvedic practitioners prescribe yoga practices as part of their health protocols. Yoga practices that incorporate Ayurvedic principles have greater therapeutic benefits.

What is Yoga?

Yoga is a vast system of knowledge and practices. It is an art and a science that has developed over thousands of years. There are many different traditions of yoga, each with its own emphasis. All traditions focus on cultivating the body, breath and mind. In each tradition, however, one of these — the body, breath or mind — is usually at center stage, with the other two being in supportive roles.

The clearest and most comprehensive description of yoga is in the *Yoga Sutras of Patanjali.* The *Yoga Sutras* are a concise description of the goals and practices of yoga. They offer practical guidelines for aligning ourselves with life's wisdom. In doing so we find ourselves being supported by life rather than being in conflict with it. It is in this alignment that we access our inherent health, wholeness and joy.

The postures (asanas) are currently the most widely practiced aspect of yoga. There are many styles of asana. One style may focus on connecting body and breath while another emphasizes musculoskeletal alignment. There are vigorous, aerobic styles of asana that heat the body, and slow, meditative styles that cool the mind. A spiritual focus might take center stage for one approach, while another is more interested in cultivating physical strength and flexibility.

One style is not inherently better than another. All have their benefits. When a particular style aligns with an individual's needs, however, it is better for them. A person with a contemplative nature might do better with a slower practice that focuses on internal awareness. A physically demanding style will give physical, action-oriented practitioners a way to focus their energy.

The numerous approaches to asana reflect the yogic wisdom that one size does *not* fit all. The practices in this book focus largely on asana, with breathwork and meditation playing a supportive role.

All yoga practitioners regardless of the style of yoga they practice or their level of experience can increase the benefits of their practice by integrating Ayurvedic principles.

What is Ayurveda?

Ayurveda is a traditional holistic medical system from India that emerged from the same philosophical ground as yoga. Dr. Vasant Lad, who introduced Ayurveda to the West, refers to Ayurveda as the "Mother of all Healing." The word Ayurveda is made up of two Sanskrit words: "ayu" meaning life, longevity and "veda" meaning knowledge or science. Thus, Ayurveda is the knowledge or science of creating health, vitality and long life.

Balance is a major theme in Ayurveda. Health, happiness and longevity are results of maintaining balance: balance in body, mind and emotions; balance in diet; balance between activity and rest; and recognizing when we are out of balance and knowing how to regain it. Balance is not static. It is an ongoing process of making adjustments as we live our lives. The art of maintaining balance is a journey in self-awareness.

The art of maintaining balance is a journey in self-awareness.

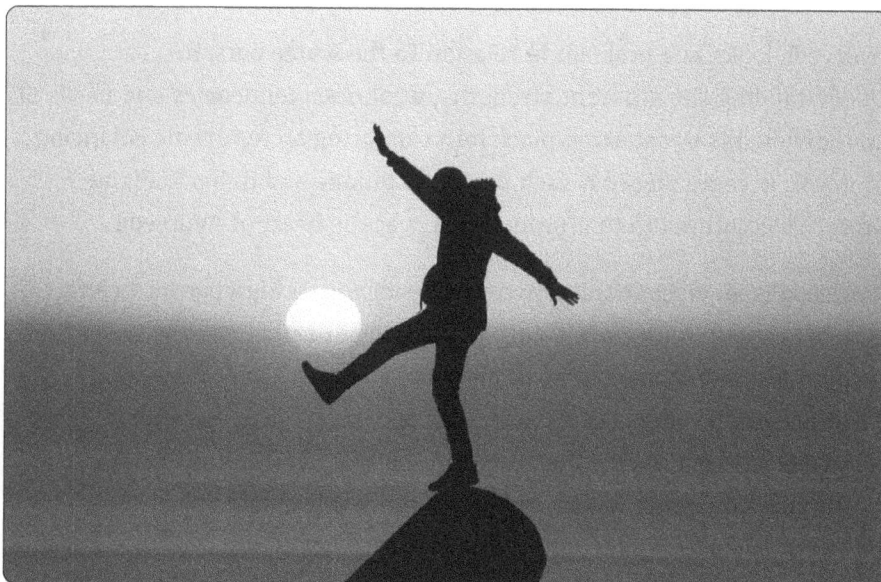

AZIZ ACHARKI | UNSPLASH

Ayurveda developed out of a close examination of nature and the recognition that we are a part of nature. We embody nature's energies and so by looking at the dynamics of balance and imbalance in nature we have a start for understanding these dynamics in ourselves. As we learn to maintain balance within ourselves and in relation to our world, we experience a spontaneous arising of health, happiness and joy.

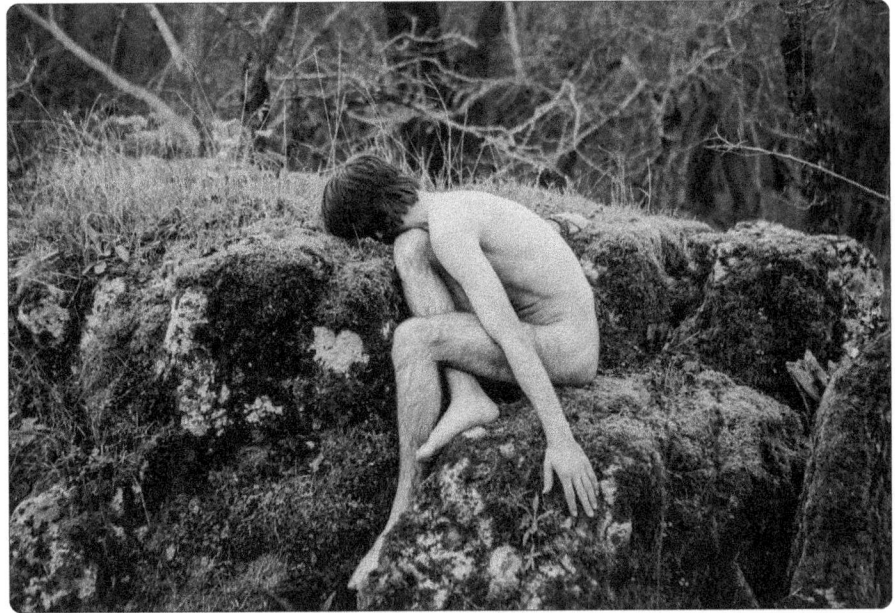

MUBARIZ MEHDIZADEH | UNSPLASH

Ayurveda looks at a problem in relation to the whole person. Understanding the different strengths, weakness, tendencies and needs of an individual is the starting place for structuring an Ayurvedic balancing protocol. Recognizing that each person is unique and individualizing protocols according to that uniqueness is at the heart of Ayurveda.

Ayurveda is an elegant and practical system with a high bar for health. It is not content with the absence of disease but rather has the goal of helping people achieve their full potential for health and happiness. Ayurveda can be very effective for healing disease. It is, however, Ayurveda's insight into preventing disease that is of profound value in our current culture where so much suffering is created by chronic health problems.

Ayurveda Increases the Benefits of Yoga

A yoga practice must serve our needs in order for it to stay vital and relevant to us. A practice that serves us when we are healthy and strong does not serve us when we are vulnerable or ill. Different times of life require different types of practice. During times of challenge it is not uncommon for people to lose connection with their practice, even though this is the time when they most need it.

Ayurveda gives us both a way to more skillfully recognize our changing needs and the understanding to adapt our practice to meet those needs. Yoga, infused with Ayurvedic wisdom, becomes a holistic practice and gives us access to more of the therapeutic, healing potential of yoga.

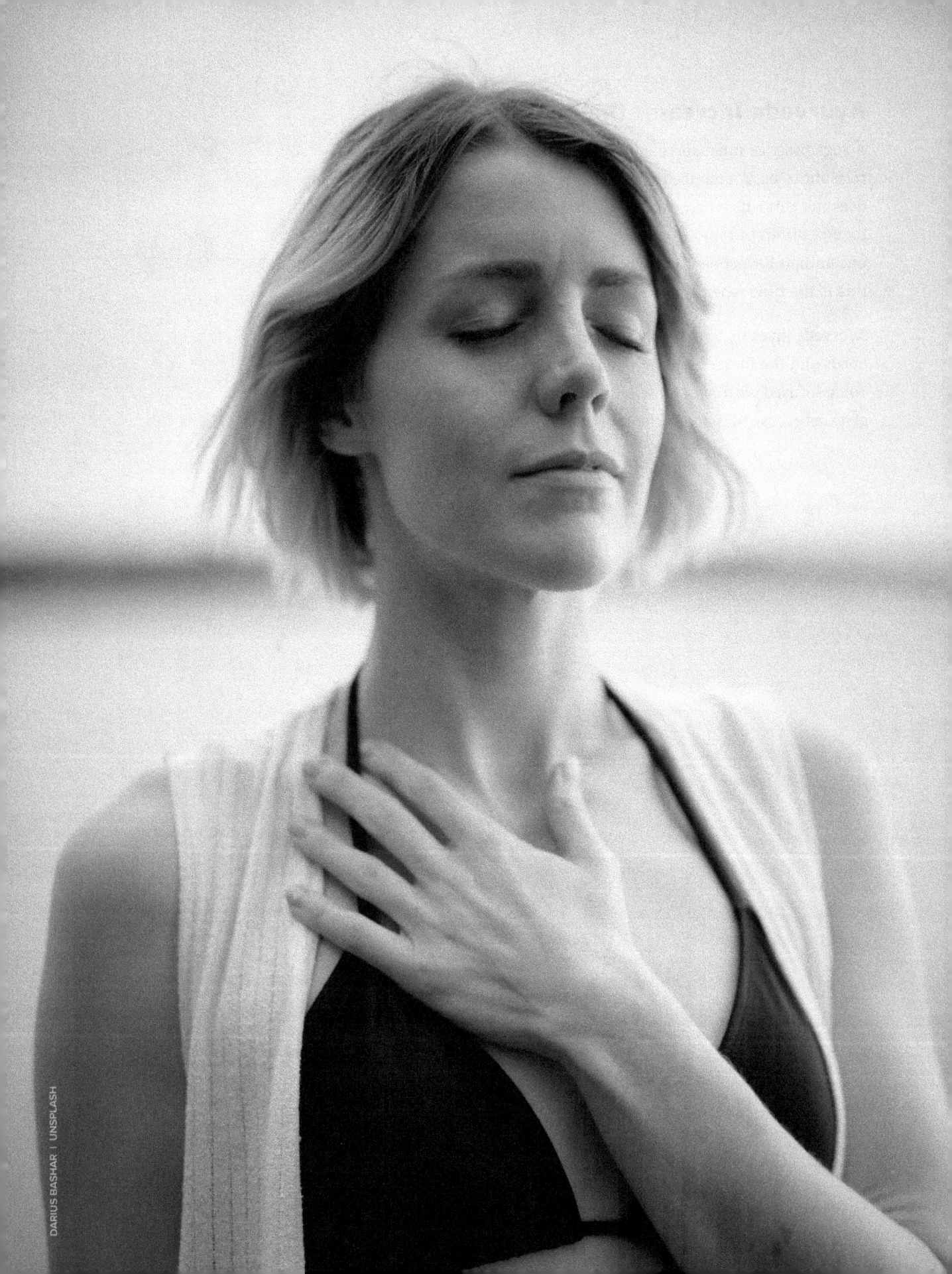

Self-Awareness and Somatic Awareness

> "Although the Greek word soma originally meant 'of the body,' it later evolved to mean the 'living body in its wholeness.' In this latter definition, soma is a process of doing and being, rather than an abstract entity. In other words, soma is a living process by which our bodily sensations, movements, perceptions, emotions and thoughts form a whole of experience."
>
> — somaticstudies.com*

Self-awareness comes in different ways. Athletes, gymnasts and people involved in other forms of physical training develop self-awareness through refining their skill. This awareness is organized around quantitative references such as how strong, how fast, how many and so on.

We also develop self-awareness in response to what our teachers, bosses and peers expect of us. This form of self-awareness develops as we try to meet their expectations. This self-awareness may feel positive or negative depending on how successful or not we are in achieving what is being asked of us.

Our culture and family send messages/images of how we should look, act and be. We internalize these messages and they become a part of how we are aware of ourselves. We may try to embody these messages/images or we may rebel against them. In either case, we develop a self-awareness in response to them.

*see Appendix, page 231

All of these types of self-awareness happen primarily in an unconscious way and are based on an external reference. In contrast, somatic awareness focuses on consciously cultivating self-awareness using internal reference. Rather than responding to an external image or goal, somatic awareness is about becoming aware of what is happening inside ourselves just as we are.

External and internal referencing enhance each other. Together they give us access to more of our potential, and a more holistic experience of ourselves.

Somatic Awareness

Somatic-Awareness Methods are the means by which we develop somatic awareness. These methods offer guidance for becoming intimate with ourselves just as we are. In these methods we are not trying to shape our selves by an idea or image. Somatic awareness methods create learning situations in which we get to know ourselves by exploring our inner world. There are no correct movements or specific outcomes that we are trying to achieve.

Somatic-Awareness Methods provide guidance for paying attention to our inner experience as part of the process of performing specific actions or movements. Our attention is directed, *not* to the doing of the movement, action, position itself, but rather to what is happening in our body while we are doing them. By paying attention to the *background* of what we are doing we are getting in touch with sensations, feeling and thoughts that are usually outside of our awareness.

Among the infinite number of things that we can explore inside of ourselves are: How are we breathing? Are we unconsciously creating tension? Are we overusing some parts of our body and underusing others? Are we accepting support from the earth? Can we do the same movement using less effort?

As we attend to ourselves in this way, the quality of the movement, action or position we are using magically improves. It is not magic, though; it is expressing the yogic notion that transformation comes through the power of awareness.

By getting in touch with ourselves through sensory-awareness processes we become more sensitive to what is happening in us physically, physiologically and psychologically. We gain the ability to influence ourselves on these levels, which gives us more control over our body, our health, and our life. While this is not magic, it can certainly feel like it.

Somatic Awareness Improves Yoga Practice

As we cultivate somatic awareness we are getting in touch with our body as it is. A major benefit of doing this is that we develop a body image that is more complete and more accurate. The more complete and more accurate is our body-image, the more skillful we can be in yoga.

An inaccurate/incomplete body-image makes us more prone to injury. It is also a significant contributor to chronic pain. We use our body based on our body-image rather than how our body actually is. When our internal image is inaccurate it is more difficult to use ourselves in a way that matches the demands of a practice. The result is that we work with our body in an imbalanced way, which stresses it and leaves us vulnerable to injury.

When we have an inaccurate body-image we also use more effort than the activity we are doing requires. We fatigue easier, and what we are doing is less enjoyable. An important part of working with somatic awareness is learning to recognize when we are using excess effort and knowing how to reduce it. Excess effort limits us in our yoga practice. It also contributes to chronic pain and the tendency toward injury. The more we are able to use the right amount of effort, the more effective and enjoyable is our practice.

History Gives Us Insight

A glance into the history of somatic awareness can enlighten us as to why it benefits us to use somatic awareness in learning Ayurveda.

The somatic awareness movement was started around a hundred years ago by four people from different countries who grappled with their respective problems. What all of these people had in common was that there was no viable solution for their problem at the time. Each, in their unique way, found a solution by paying deep, sensitive attention to what was happening inside their bodies.

F.M. Alexander was an Australian actor who began losing his voice. He resolved this problem by paying careful attention to how he moved his neck and head as he began to speak.

Elsa Gindler was a German gymnastics teacher. She contracted tuberculosis but couldn't afford to go to a sanatorium for treatment. In turning her attention inward she not only was able to access her capacity for rejuvenation, but she taught herself how to breathe in one lung so the other lung could rest and heal.

Gerda Alexander was born in Germany and moved to Denmark as a young woman. In dealing with rheumatic fever and endocarditis, her background in performing arts and movement led her to focus her attention inward to find a way of moving her body that would support her healing.

Moshe Feldenkrais was born in Russia and as a teenager moved to Palestine. A knee injury from soccer haunted him for many years. Feldenkrais used his education as a physicist, engineer and black belt in judo to begin a deep somatic inquiry into the relationship between how he moved and his knee problem.

All of these people resolved their problem through developing refined awareness of what was happening inside their bodies. They all, in their different ways, cultivated somatic awareness and left a legacy of a well-developed method for cultivating somatic awareness.

Ayurveda is a holistic system. Accessing the maximum benefit of Ayurveda using yoga happens most easily when we use whole-person learning, which means using both mental/cognitive and sensory/embodied learning. The practices offered in this book are presented as somatic-awareness explorations using Ayurvedic focuses. They are designed for helping people develop an embodied, experiential understanding of Ayurveda. Learning about Ayurveda with somatic awareness couples the healing wisdom of Ayurveda with the healing benefits of somatic awareness. Through somatic awareness we embody Ayurvedic principles and know them as living realities in our own body.

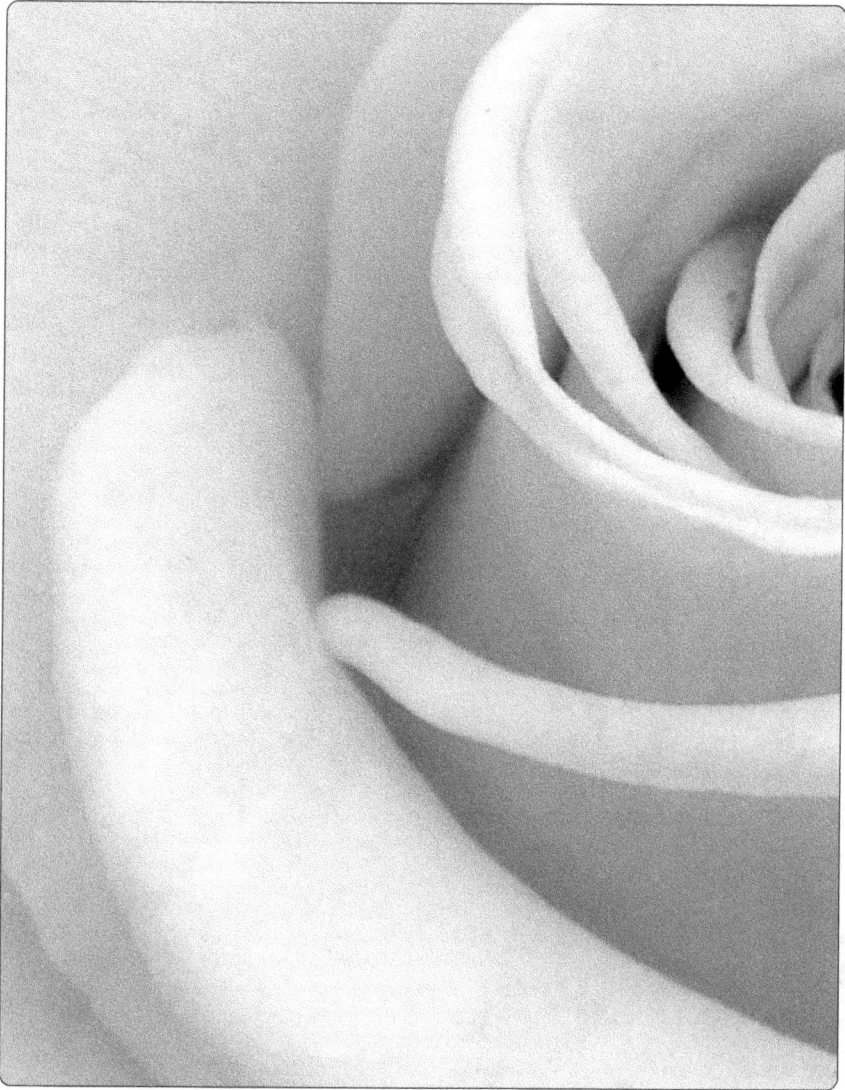

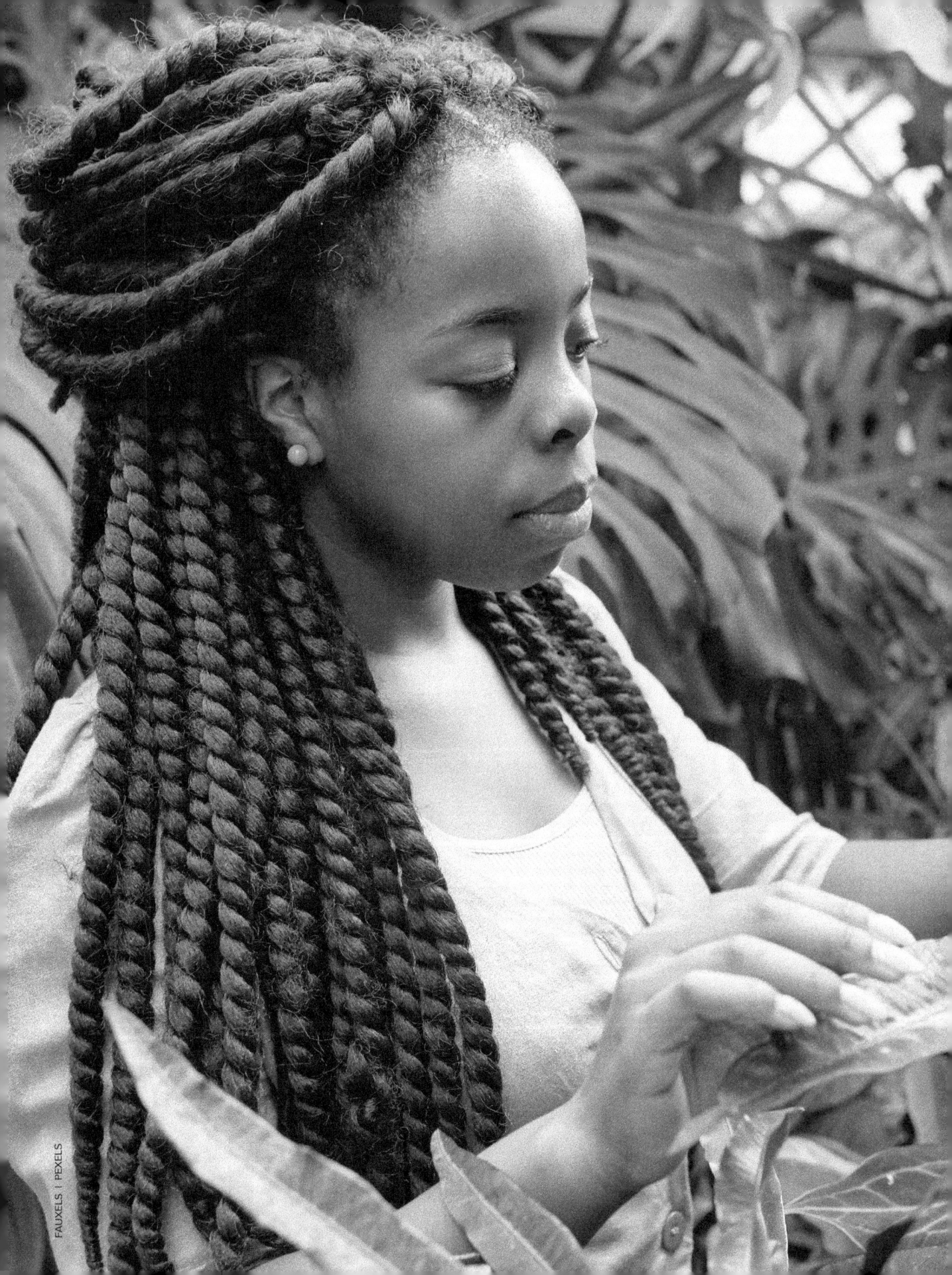

Part ONE

Ayurvedic Anatomy & Physiology

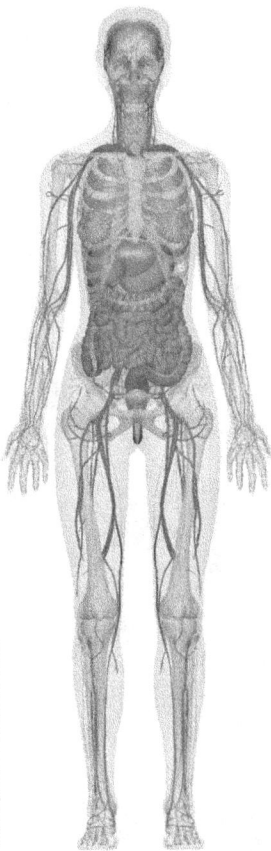

The above image represents the Western view of anatomy, while the image to the right represents Eastern energetic anatomy.

The Basics of Ayurvedic Anatomy & Physiology

A few months into my Ayurvedic training

I started feeling frustrated because I knew I was missing some key piece of understanding. I didn't know what it was, of course, so I was awkward in trying to ask about it. I kept trying to ask, however, and my frustration continued to increase when I did not get an answer that satisfied me. One day out of his own frustration with me my teacher blurted out, *"This is nothing more than Ayurvedic anatomy and physiology."*

The light bulb went on for me! That was the answer I needed. Western anatomy and physiology had greatly informed my practice and teaching of yoga. A slight adjustment in my thinking made it easy to exchange western anatomy and physiology for its Ayurvedic counter-part. All of the information and exotic names I had been learning suddenly became practical. A whole new understanding of Ayurveda popped open for me.

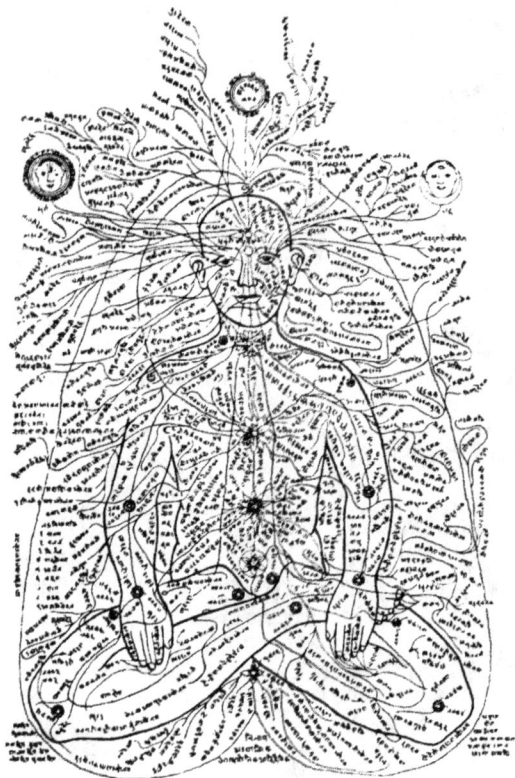

Three basic principles of Ayurvedic anatomy and physiology are covered in this book. They are **the five elements, the three doshas, the five pranas.**

The five elements — earth, water, fire, air and space — compose the primordial energy/matter out of which everything in the universe is created. Everything in our world, including our bodies, is an interplay of the different qualities and dynamics of this energy/matter. Since we are created from the elements, exploring the elements and their qualities is a way of getting to know ourselves.

Doshas are Ayurveda's way of looking at how the five elements function in our body. Each dosha is made up of two elements. Ayurvedic healing principles are based on the understanding of the doshas and how they express in our body, mind and emotions. Balancing the doshas is the goal of Ayurveda. Balanced doshas are synonymous with good health; imbalanced doshas are synonymous with reduced health and disease.

At the heart of Ayurveda is recognizing when and in what way the doshas are out of balance, and knowing how to restore their balance. An Ayurvedic doctor approaches a patient with the goal of doshic balance in mind. The process outlined in this book is a self-care version of this same goal.

Prana is the vital energy of our body, and it is the life-force within our every cell, tissue and organ. Prana is intimately related to the breath. Prana moves through our body as five directions of flow. Each direction of flow supports the structures and functions of the area of the body through which it moves. Working with the five pranas is a simple and potent way to apply Ayurveda to the practice of yoga.

The three doshas and the five pranas all arise from the elements. A dosha is a combination of two elements, and prana is a subtle aspect of the air element. Once we become aware of the elements, doshas and pranas in our own body, they can easily be integrated in the practice of yoga.

THE ELEMENTS
- Earth
- Water
- Fire
- Air
- Space

THE DOSHAS
- Vata
- Pitta
- Kapha

THE PRANAS
- Prana
- Samana
- Apana
- Udana
- Vyana

What Are the Elements?

Yoga and Ayurveda see life as an
expression of five elemental *energies:*
earth, water, fire, air and space.
*It is from these elemental energies that
the elements of our natural world arise.*

Understanding the elements and how they function in the human body
is the foundation for understanding Ayurveda. Getting to know ourselves
through this elemental perspective is how we start applying Ayurveda
to yoga.

Simply by being alive we are in touch with the energies of the elements.
We know that earth is solid and that water flows. We know that fire is
hot, air can move and that everything is held within space. Ayurveda has
refined and expanded this awareness of the elements, applied it to the
understanding of human life, and codified it into an elegant, holistic
system for creating health and wellness.

We begin our exploration of the elements with a contemplative journey
of the elemental dynamics in nature.

We then turn our attention to each individual element and its meaning
for us.

At the end of the discussion of each element there is guided process for
getting in touch with the element in your own body.

Entering Our Elemental World

We will enter into our elemental world through a journey of the imagination.

Viewing it from the perspective of an astronaut, we see our living earth as being composed of inter-acting elements that are constantly changing, that are constantly going in and out of balance.

This is a solid step in understanding Ayurveda and how it can be applied to yoga practice. Read the words on the following pages slowly, with meditative awareness, so the images presented have time to soak into your body/mind as a felt sense.

SAMUEL SILITONGA / PEXELS

CONTEMPLATING OUR ELEMENTAL WORLD

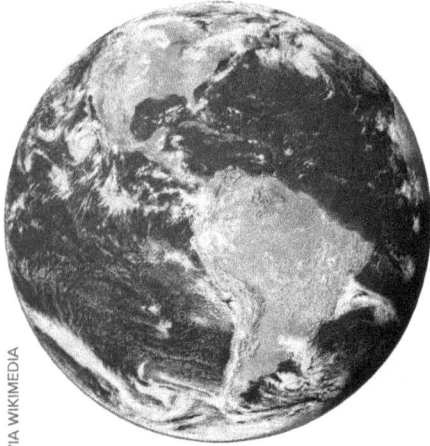

Imagine that you are relaxing in outer space and getting to know our world from that viewpoint.

Open your gaze and take in the limitless black space around you.

Turn your attention to the world we live on, a stunningly beautiful, multi-colored globe suspended in that limitless black space.

Air surrounds our planet in a protective embrace. The hot light of the sun and the cool light of the moon take turns bathing it with their light.

Vast expanses of water cover most of world's surface, coloring it with many shades of blue. Juxtaposing these layers of blue are large masses of land colored with infinite shades of brown, green and gold.

Coming in closer to the earth, more and more details emerge.

Lakes appear as blue dots of various shapes and sizes. Rivers and streams carve straight and curved lines through the land as they flow toward their ultimate home in the vast blue oceans.

Trees express themselves in a wide variety of sizes, shapes and shades of green. Craggy mountains, gentle hills, wind-shaped deserts and softly-colored plains contribute their colors and textures.

Sitting in the presence of the living beauty of this planet, the elemental energies come into your awareness.

ELEMENTS

The earth element gives our planet substance and stability, water provides it with moisture, and the sun's fire gives it warmth, while air caresses everything on its surface, and space offers itself as the container for it all.

When these elemental energies are in balance, days are calm and peaceful.

When one or more elements increase, life is disturbed. Sun that is too hot can ignite a forest fire, dry up the water and create a drought, or send people to the hospital with heatstroke. In excess, water can flood the banks of a river and carry away houses. Overly activated air can become a tornado that levels everything in its path or it can whip the ocean water into a hurricane that strips the land and dissolves the foundation of a city. Even our seemingly reliable earth can break apart with an earthquake, laying waste to everything it once supported.

These disturbances pass, the elements return to balance and we again experience the calm of a balanced world.

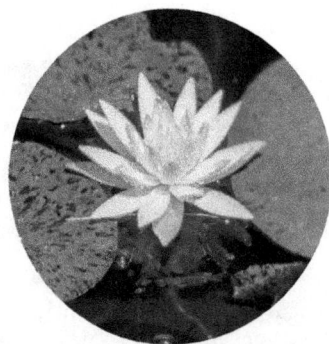

Close your eyes for a few moments
and contemplate the world as an interplay of elements.
Contemplate also that you emerged from this world —
and you too are an expression of these elemental energies.

The World Is Us

We are a smaller version of this world and its elements. We are fashioned from the same five elements and are prone to the same elemental imbalances. These imbalances express in us on the mental and emotional, as well as the physical level.

We intuitively recognize our elemental nature and express that recognition in phrases like: "He is so *grounded,*" or "They are an *earthy* couple," "She is an *air*-head," or "I am feeling *spacey* today." We may feel stung by someone's *fiery* temper or frustrated by somebody's *wishy-washy* personality.

In Ayurveda, a small imbalance in our internal elements is seen as the seed of a health problem. When we do end up with a health problem or disease, it is viewed as an elemental imbalance that was left unchecked and so became bigger, stronger and more complex. Recognizing small elemental imbalances and intervening in order to regain balance is how we keep ourselves healthy and well.

In learning about the elements, we are learning about ourselves. Elemental energies are our energies. In the following chapters we will get to know each of the elements and how they function in our body.

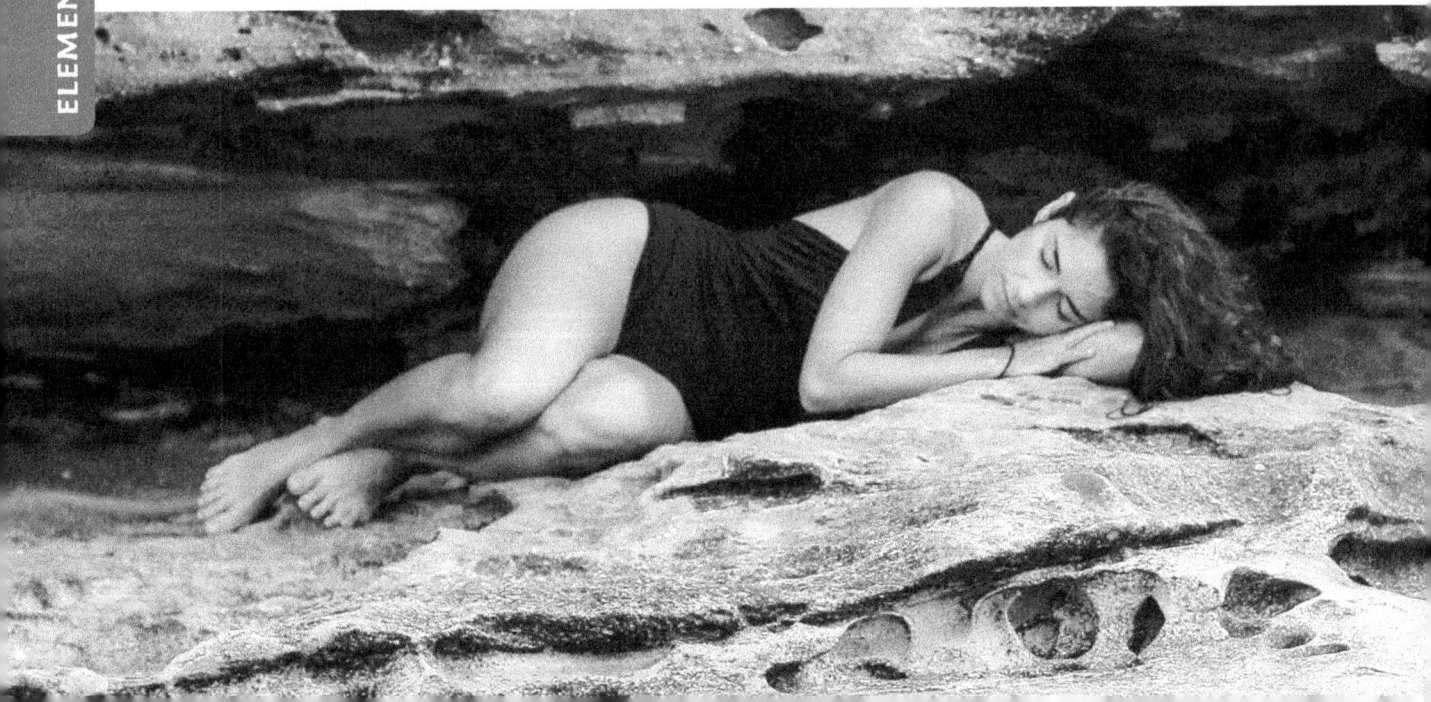

Reflections on the External Elements and Their Counterparts in You

- Let the water of your morning shower resonate with the more than seventy percent water that is your body.

- While drinking a glass of water be aware of it merging with your internal water in the way a river merges with the ocean.

- When cooking food, momentarily contemplate your stomach as a "pot" where the heat of your digestive fire "cooks" the food for your body.

- Contemplate the kinship that your internal heat has with the sun.

- Feel the movement of a breeze resonating with the movement of air as it flows in and out of your lungs.

- When you see weeds crowding out flowers in a garden, reflect on how excess thoughts and emotions crowd out the more subtle experiences of peace and contentment. Remember how everything needs sufficient space to live and grow.

- As you gaze into space, reflect on the spaces in your body; such as the space in your sinuses, in your windpipe and in your intestines.

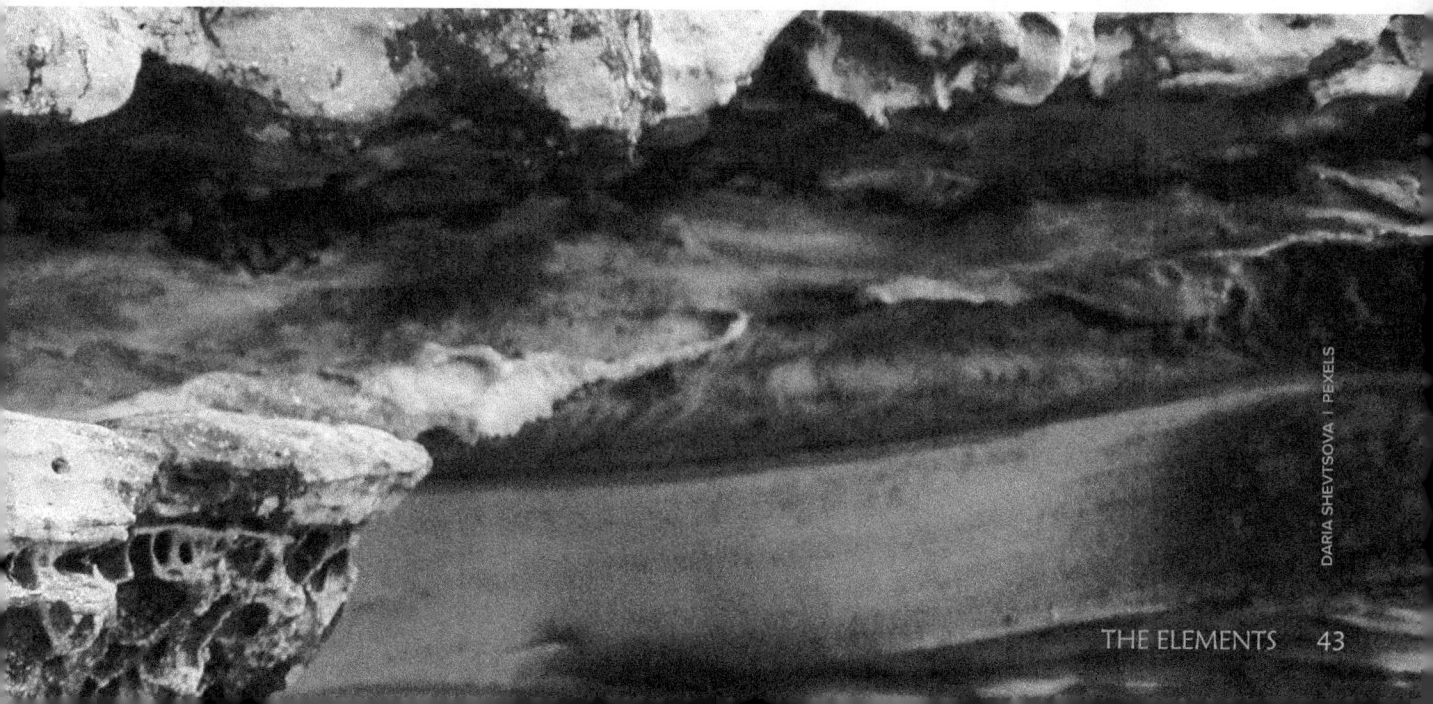

DARIA SHEVTSOVA | PEXELS

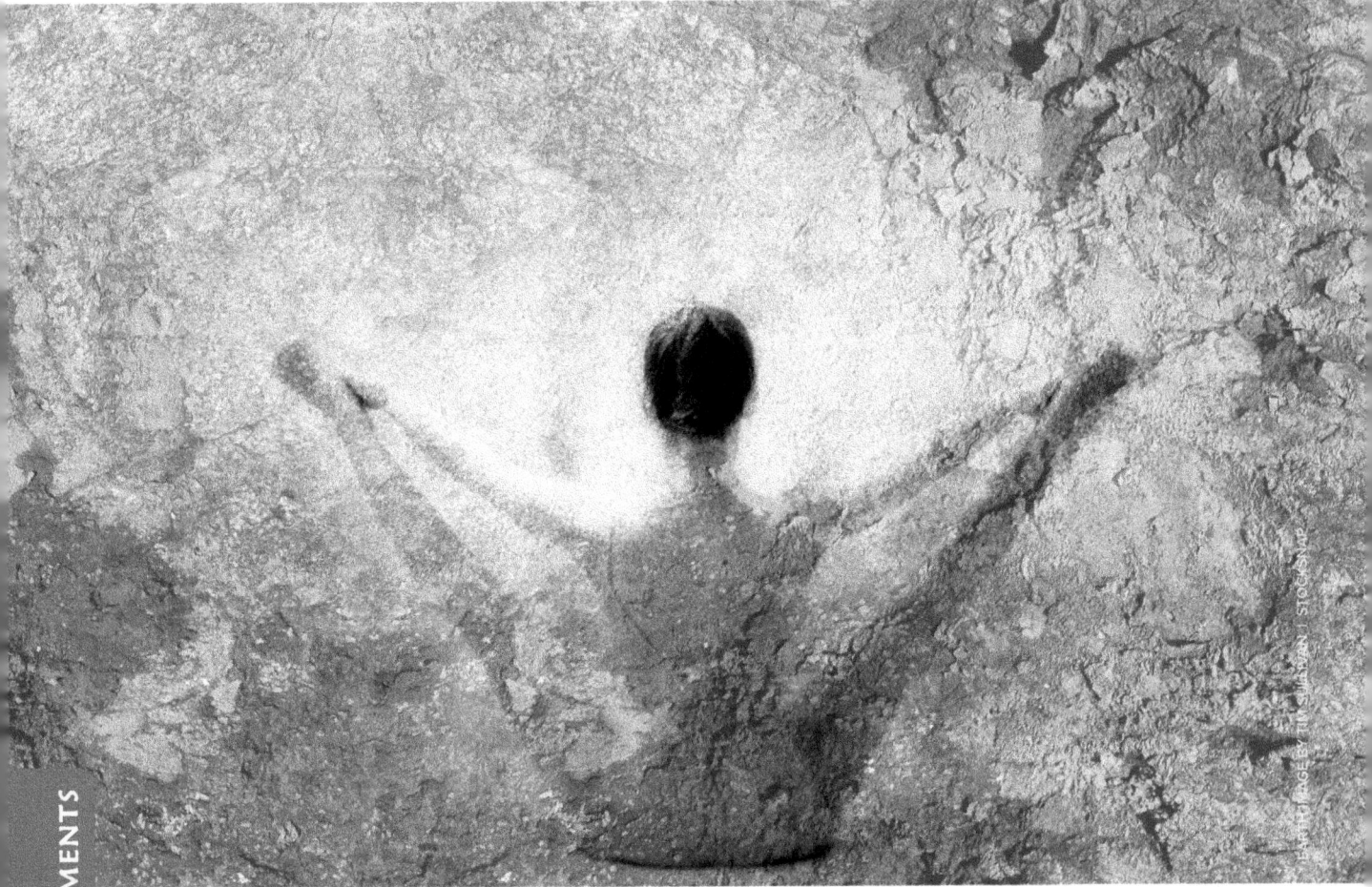

ELEMENTS

Let us thank the Earth
That offers ground for home
And holds our feet firm
— John O'Donohue

The Elements - Earth

The earth element is the substance of our body.

Earth is heavy and solid. When we feel the weight of our body, we are feeling the heaviness and solidity of our earth element. Earth is difficult to move. Just think about the effort needed to dig a hole in the ground or distribute a load of soil through your yard. The earth in our body is also not easily moved.

When we are feeling tossed around by life, we can center ourselves by connecting to the heaviness and solidity of our body, which is another way of staying connecting to our earth. When we are depleted, turning our attention to earth gives us access to the stillness we need to rest deeply. If our mind and emotions are agitated, we can pacify them by tuning into and feeling our body/earth.

Earth needs to be loosened if it is to be fruitful. This is as true for the earth of our body as it is for the earth in our garden. In growing a garden, we must loosen the earth so the seeds that we plant can take root and grow. In *loosening* our body with asana, we are creating a vital and responsive body capable of supporting us in growing our lives.

Earth is balanced when it is in proper relationship to the other elements. Excess earth in our body creates excess heaviness in our body. The heaviness of excess earth dulls the other elements. On the contrary, balanced earth helps to keep the other elements in balance. Asana practice, in keeping our earth balanced, supports balance in all of the elements.

When our internal earth is balanced, we are confident, patient and content. We have the steadiness to stand strong in the face of life's challenges.

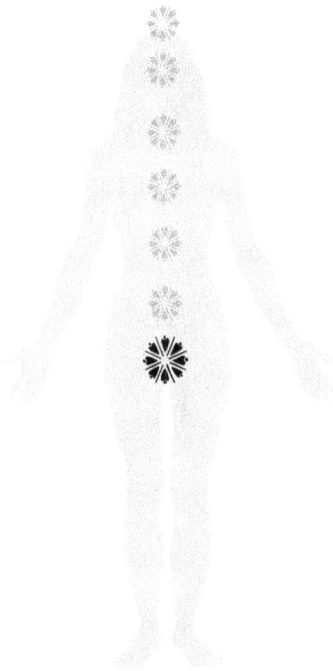

The earth element is related to the **1st chakra**. *Lam* is the seed mantra of the 1st chakra. Focusing on the 1st chakra and the *lam* mantra during asana or meditation contribute to balanced earth. You can also use the first chakra or *lam* as earth-balancing touchstones during daily activities. (See Appendix on page 227 for more on how to use chakras and seed mantras.)

Excess Earth and How to Balance it.

Earth is gravity bound. Earth has no inherent capacity to move, so when we become *earth-bound* with excess earth, we lose touch with our lightness and ease.

Too much earth smothers our enthusiasm and makes it difficult to connect with life's joy. Excess earth makes us prone to dullness and depression. This lethargy and depression can prevent us from accessing the *oomph* we need to exercise, and without exercise earth tends to go farther out of balance and we are vulnerable to health problems.

Earth affects and is affected by the other elements. Excess earth leaves us not only vulnerable to earth-related problems but also to problems related to the other elements. For example, fire is the elemental energy involved in digesting our food. Excess earth can smother our internal fire, and so weaken our digestion.

When we feel bogged down under the weight of excess earth, our first step in moving out from under it is making a decision to do so. Under the weight of excess earth, making *any* decision is not easy, particularly a decision to mobilize ourselves when we feel weighted down. Making this decision, however, is the necessary first step.

After we have decided we are going to find our vitality and mobilize our earth, we can then engage the elemental energies of air and fire. Engaging the heat of fire helps us to warm and penetrate our earth/body to make it more malleable. In awakening our fire we are also increasing our vitality. Engaging air is a means of lightening, aerating and mobilizing our earth, and gaining access to lightheartedness and physical mobility.

1ST CHAKRA

Element: Earth
Seed mantra: *Lam*

(The "a" in all the seed sounds is pronounced as in "some.")

ELEMENTS

Vigorous asanas such as standing poses and inversions are good for generating heat/fire, as are heating pranayamas such as Bastrika and Kapalabhati.* The continuous movement of vinyasas, whether gentle or vigorous, awakens the air element. Vigorous vinyasas have the added benefit of also stimulating the fire element.

Activating fire and air energies together will more quickly reduce the heavy, static and dull energies of excess earth. If we try to engage fire and air before we are ready, however, the weight of excess earth might be too much for us and we end up being discouraged. This is a familiar scenario for most of us in starting something with great enthusiasm only to become unable to sustain it. We are more likely to be able to sustain fire- and air-inspired asana if we start small and build gradually.

If we don't have the physical or emotional energy to engage fire and air, we can look toward the water element. Engaging water energy allows us to mobilize and enliven our earth/body more gradually. Doing a number of gentle seated or reclining poses with short holds is an easy way to start moving our earth/body. We can tease ourselves into longer and stronger holds until we are able to meet the challenge of more vigorous standing and inverted poses. We can think of this process as similar to soaking the heavy earth of our body with water so it becomes more malleable and responsive.

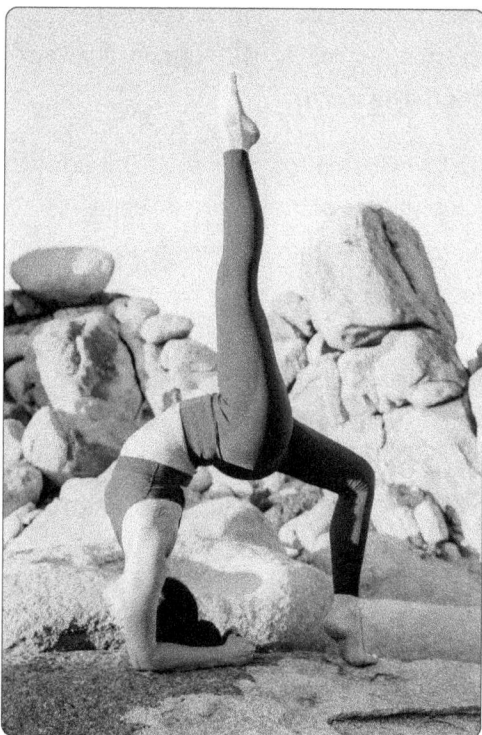

WESLEY TINGEY | UNSPLASH

see Appendix, page 228

Strengthen Weak Earth

When our earth element is weak, we are *ungrounded* and our body is unstable. Weak earth leaves us prone to illness and injury.

Restorative asanas are a good starting place for moving toward balanced earth. We can also use reclining asanas to develop some stability and strength as a way to transition into more challenging asanas. My favorite way of strengthening earth when I am depleted is doing a series of reclining asanas in which each asana is followed by savasana. If our earth element is very weak it is important to go slowly in rebuilding it.

An easy support for awakening earth is simply being in nature. When we are in nature our body's earth resonates with our planet's earth and our body/earth remembers how to be in balance. Doing asana in nature is wonderfully earth-balancing.

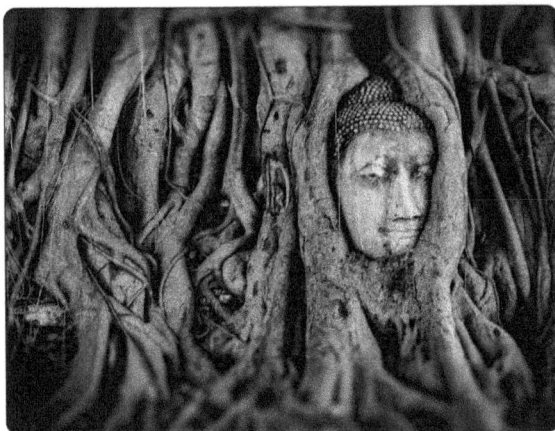

WALKERSSK | PIXABAY

Imagination is also very effective for bringing balancing energies into our practice. We can imagine being in nature and absorbing nature's energy into our body while doing a practice. Or, we can imagine roots growing down from our pelvis, through our legs and deep into the earth.

Feeling connected to our body is important for keeping our earth balanced. Regular asana practice is the obvious go-to for *working* with our body, but asana does not automatically give us a sense of *connection* to our body. Doing asana with attention on sensing the body will develop that connection. Doing asana with an athletic focus can result in objectifying the body, which disallows that connection. We can enjoy an athletic focus and create a connection to our body by, after every asana practice, doing a deep Savasana and fully sensing the body with an attitude of appreciation.

ELEMENTS

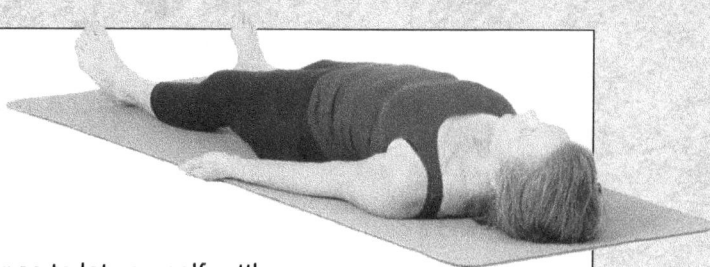

Awakening Prana ~ Savasana and Crocodile

🕐 8 - 12 minutes

◎ Lie on your back and take a minute or so to let yourself settle.

◎ Sense the contact of your body on the floor and let go into that support.

◎ Let your awareness descend through your back body and move a foot or so into the earth. Rest in and breathe with your connection to the earth.

◎ Take a luxurious amount of time to enjoy connecting to and breathing with the earth.

◎ Let your awareness descend another foot into the earth and repeat the process.

◎ Roll very slowly, heavily and lazily onto your stomach. As you roll, feel the weight of your body and maintain your sense of connection to the earth.

◎ Rest on your stomach for a minute or so until your body, mind and breath have settled into the position.

◎ Let your awareness descend through your front body and move a foot or so into the earth. Rest in and breathe with your connection to the earth.

◎ Take a luxurious amount of time to enjoy connecting to and breathing with the earth.

◎ Let your awareness descend another foot into the earth and repeat the process.

◎ Finish by resting for a minute or so on your stomach or back, sensing the weight of your body.

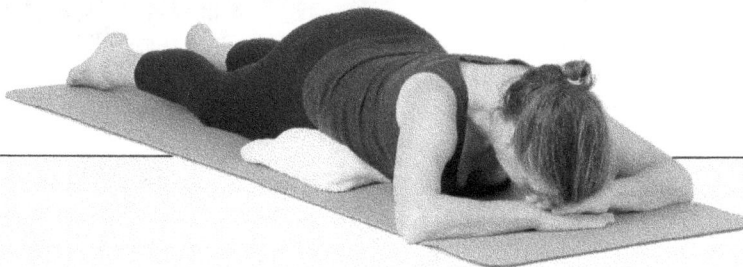

1st Chakra and Seed Mantra Meditation

🕐 8 - 10 minutes

◎ Find a comfortable sitting position.

◎ Take a few minutes to let your mind, body and breath settle.

◎ Bring your awareness to the pelvic floor in the area of the tailbone; breathe gently as if breathing in and out through this area. Continue in this way for a few minutes.

◎ Continue breathing in and out through the area around the tailbone and, on the exhalation, begin to repeat the seed mantra *lam*. You can repeat the mantra either vocally or mentally, or you can alternate between mental and vocalized repetitions. Allow the vibration of the mantra to soak into the 1st chakra.

◎ Finish with a few moments of rest.

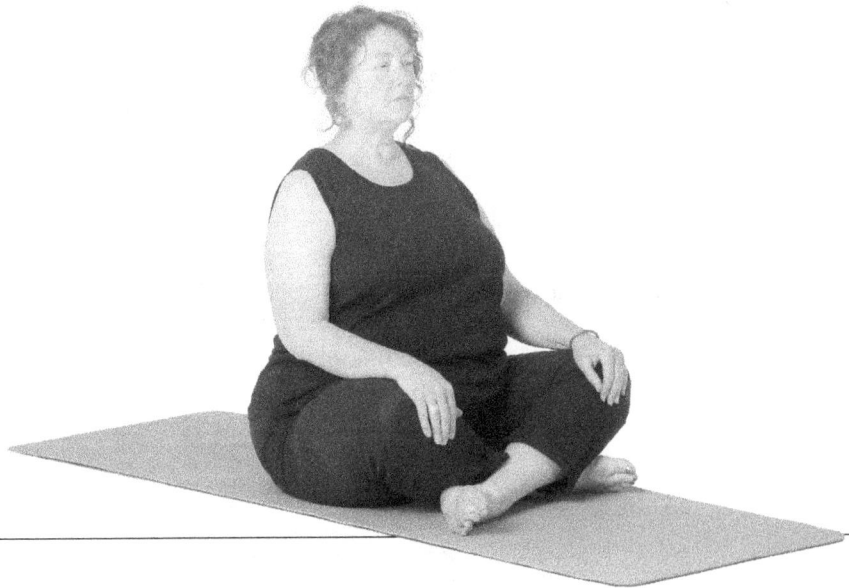

ELEMENTS

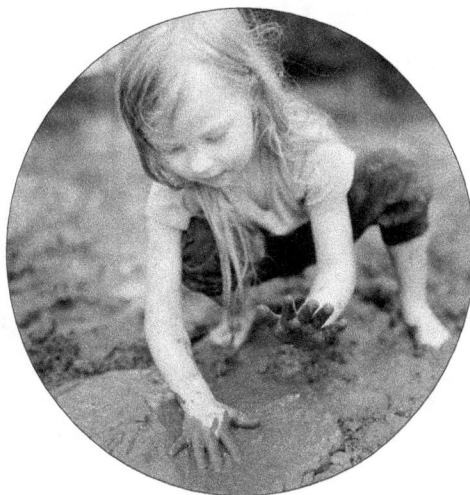

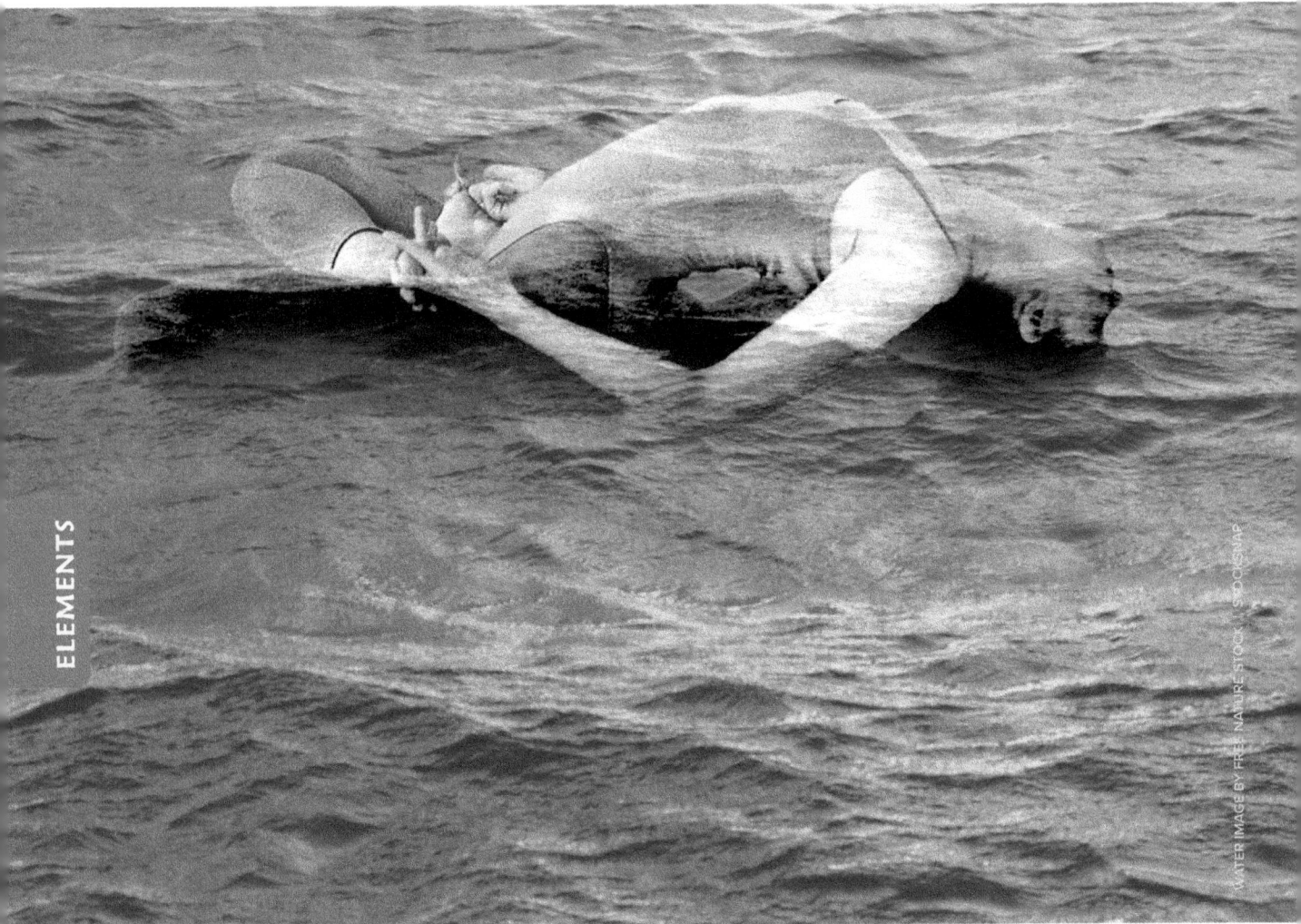

Blessed be Water,
Our first mother.
— John O'Donohue

WATER IMAGE BY FREE-NATURE-STOCK, STOCKSNAP

ELEMENTS

• EARTH   • **WATER**   • FIRE   • AIR   • SPACE

The Elements - Water

The fluid aspect of our body comes from the water element. Every cell, tissue and organ in our body is surrounded by and suspended in fluidity.

The rhythmic ebb and flow of these fluids underlies the cleansing and nourishing actions that keep our body alive. Getting in touch with our fluid aspect gives us a soft yet powerful strength in both body and mind.

The brain and spinal cord float in and are protected by cerebrospinal fluid. Synovial fluid lubricates and protects our joints so we can move without pain. Blood carries nourishment to our cells and removes the waste products created by cellular activity.

Water cools, moistens, coheres, soothes, softens, and spreads. These qualities support integration in our body, mind and emotions. It is through the water element that we experience a sense of wholeness.

Our internal organs are largely fluid. Awareness of them as fluid weight makes them a valuable resource in asana practice. Sensing our organs as bags of water that can be compressed, shaped and shifted in different directions allows us to use them to support musculoskeletal actions. We can also use our organs in this way to open spaces in our body and so create more freedom of movement. Entering into an asana by initiating from the organs rather than from the limbs gives us a quiet, cohesive, organic strength.

Water, like earth, is under the control of gravity. Water either pools or flows downward. Its gravity-bound, fluid nature makes it a valuable energy to engage for soothing our body/mind, softening hard emotions or releasing tension. Sensing our watery aspect allows us to connect with its buoyancy and to use that buoyancy for creating ease in asana. Accessing our fluid nature in asana brings a sense of pleasurable connectedness.

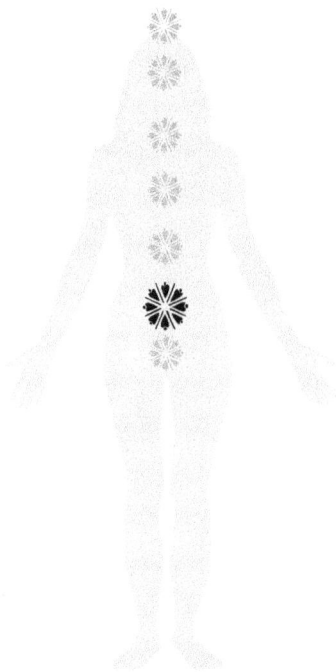

The water element is related to the **2nd chakra**. The seed mantra of the 2nd chakra is *vam*. Focusing on the 2nd chakra and repeating *vam* during asana or meditation contribute to balancing our water element. These focuses can also be used during daily activities as earth-balancing touchstones. (See Appendix on page 227 for more on how to use chakras and seed mantras.)

Too Much or Too Little Water

With excess water we become too *watery. Wateriness* can express mentally, emotionally or physically. A watery mental state shows up as unclear thinking and difficulty in making decisions. We don't know how to stand firm in relationship to ourselves, to ideas or to our world. Excess water can leave us unmoored and floating through our days.

Emotionally, excess water expresses in being clingy, apathetic or excessively emotional. It can make us prone to being overly influenced by people, advertising or fads. Standing up for ourselves or standing solidly in a position is challenging.

Physically, excess water can express as sloppiness or instability. Swelling and congestion, such as swollen ankles and lung or sinus congestion, are expressions of excess water. Excess water can also create poor digestion by dampening down our digestive fire.

When we have a deficiency in the water element, we are *dry*. Dryness withers the body and expresses as thinning tissues, muscular stiffness and/or constipation. The body loses its cohesiveness and plumpness, becoming brittle. Too little water, like too much water, reduces the effectiveness of our digestion.

Emotionally, too little water leaves us unable to connect to people, nature and our world. We lose access to the life-juice of creativity and play. Mental dryness robs us of inspiration and imagination and so narrows our thinking and shrinks our life.

2ND CHAKRA

Element: Water
Seed mantra: *Vam*

Maintaining Balanced Water

When our water element is balanced, we feel cohesive and *together*. Balanced water supports us in feeling connected to ourselves, our community and to life. This in turn supports feelings of satisfaction and contentment.

Our internal waters need to flow freely, and they need to be contained. Any well-structured asana practice helps us develop muscular-skeletal integration, massages our internal organs and washes away tension. These are all necessary components of maintaining balance between containment and free-flow.

Since water is gravity bound, activities that are *up-lifting* and vitalizing are useful for keeping our internal water balanced. Under the influence of gravity, the fluids in our body can pool in the lower body. This creates suboptimal blood flow to the heart and brain thus leaving them undernourished.

Inversions allow fluids from the lower body to flow to the heart and brain, thus nourishing these vital organs. Someone who cannot comfortably sustain inversions can get the same benefits with supported inversions such as half shoulder stand with legs resting on the wall.

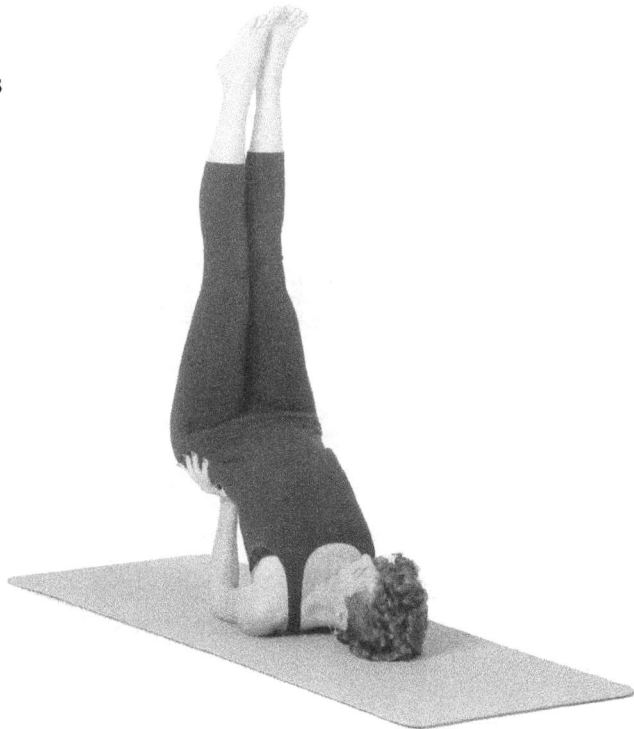

Elemental Support for Balancing Water

Fire stimulates water. A vigorous asana practice with long holds is heating and so awakens the fire element. The heat enlivens our inner water and allows it to flow more easily. Heating pranayamas such as Bastrika and Kapalabhati* can also be used to stimulate fire.

A sharp mental focus helps to balance the water element. Sharpness is a dynamic of fire and a sharp focus stimulates fire. It can be difficult for someone with excess water to sustain a sharp focus for very long, so it is better that they start with a short practice time and slowly increase it. A shorter amount of time with a sharp focus is better than a longer period time with a dull focus.

Spending a few minutes concentrating on the tip of a candle flame is a good way to cultivate a sharp focus.

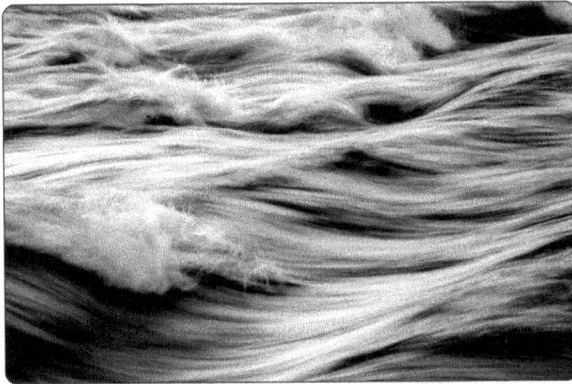

Air energy can be used to mobilize water and awaken it out of a stagnant state. The simplest and most effective way to engage air is through the practice of vinyasas. The Sun Salutation is a vinyasa that most people know.

Any variation of the Sun Salutation done for 30-45 minutes works well for balancing water.

If that length of time seems long to you, focus on finding a comfortable rhythm. With a good rhythm, a forty-minute Sun Salutation is no different than going for a walk of the same duration. Of course, you want to start with a length of time that you can do without strain and gradually add minutes.

A series of asanas with short holds is also useful for mobilizing water.

see Appendix, page 228

Child's Pose with Breath Awareness

🕐 5 or 6 minutes

༄ Come into **Child's Pose** with a folded towel between your belly and thighs. Use a large enough towel so your belly is in full contact with the towel. Make any adjustments you need to be comfortable. Your arms can rest alongside your legs or extend forward on the floor above your head.

༄ Turn your awareness to the contact of your belly with the towel. Sense your breathing, noticing how the inhalation and exhalation create an alternating increasing-and-decreasing pressure between your belly and the towel.

༄ Notice that each breath is subtly different. Relax into the rhythm of your breathing and sense its subtle wave-like motion.

༄ Leisurely alternate your awareness between the sensations that the movement of your breathing creates through your whole body, and the increasing-and-decreasing pressure your breathing creates between the contact of your belly and the towel.

༄ Rest for a minute or more on your back.

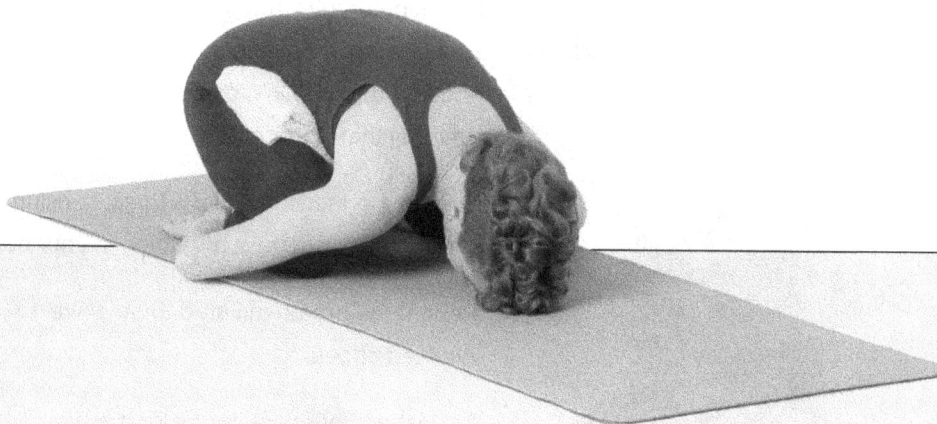

Breath-Initiated Torso Wave

🕐 5 - 7 minutes

≈ Take a comfortable seated position with your palms resting on your belly. Sense the in-and-out movement of your breathing. Bring your awareness to your abdomen and sense the in-and-out movement of your breathing.

≈ Let the movement of your breathing initiate a small wave-like movement in the torso. Waves can move in any direction so explore which direction a wave most easily happens. Give time for this movement to grow naturally. Inspire yourself in the movement by bringing to mind gentle waves in water.

≈ The movement can start out tiny. It may not even be noticeable to someone watching you. Once a movement arises naturally, it can unfold into a movement of your whole torso. Evoking a body memory of floating in water or lying by the seashore and letting the waves lap on your body can also help awaken your torso to fluid movement.

The size of the movement is not important. The important thing is that the movement has a soft, organic wave-like quality. Some people find this kind of movement easy and natural while others find it awkward. If you are the latter, just be patient. Remember that your body is mostly water and give yourself some time to let that water express itself in movement.

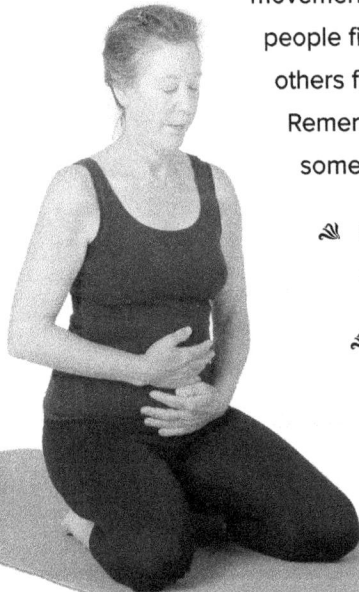

≈ Rest for a short time in **Child's Pose**, sensing the wave-like motion of your breathing in your belly.

≈ Repeat the breath-initiated torso wave outlined above.

≈ Rest on your back for as long as you like.

Second Chakra Seed Mantra Meditation

🕐 7 - 10 minutes

⬩ Find a comfortable seated position.

⬩ Take a few minutes to settle yourself.

⬩ Bring your awareness to a point two inches below the navel near the front of the spine.

⬩ Breathe gently as if the breath is moving in and out through this point.

⬩ When your body and breath have relaxed into this focus, begin to repeat the seed mantra *vam* either vocally or mentally, filling this chakra point with the vibration of *vam*.

⬩ Finish by resting quietly for a minute or so.

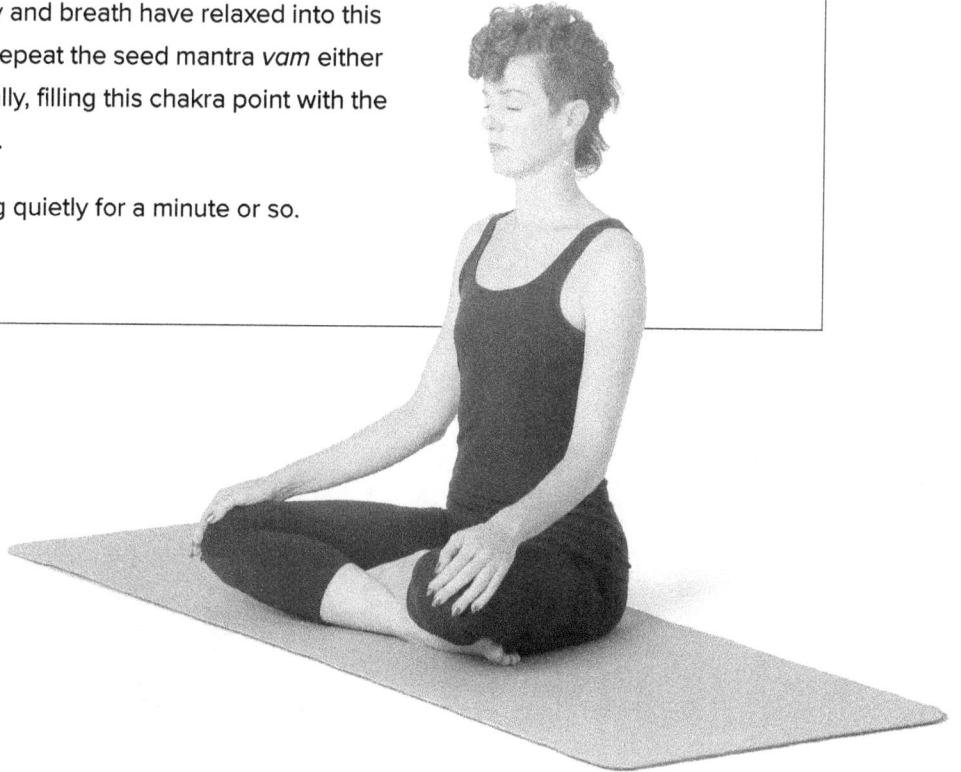

Praise the pure presence of Fire
That burns from within.
— *John O'Donohue*

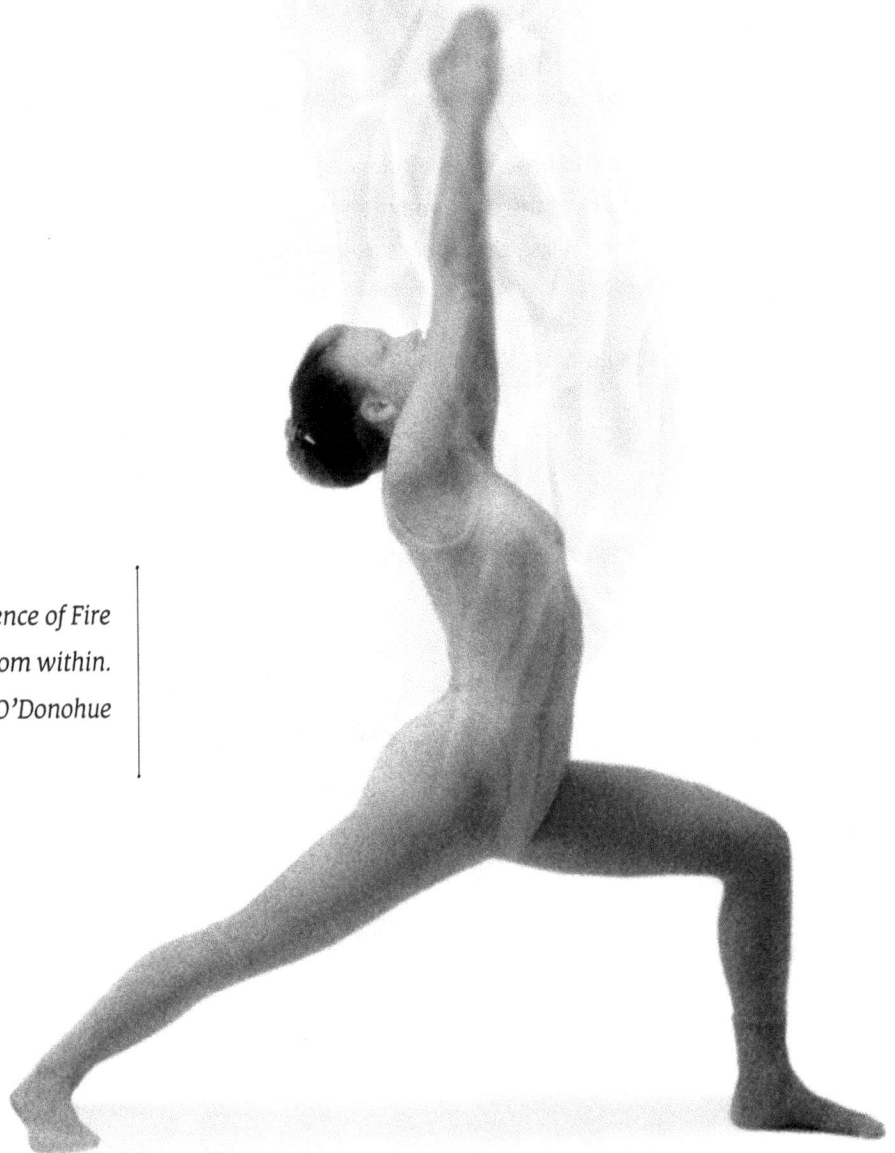

The Elements - Fire

Just as the sun gives heat and light to the earth, so, too, our internal fire gives heat and light to our body.

When our internal fire is healthy it expresses through us as bright eyes, luminous skin and radiance of being.

Fire is our digestive power. The transforming power of fire gives us energy and vitality. Fire processes the food we eat, converts it into a form that our body can use, and then further converts it into energy.

Everything that we take into ourselves from the outside world must be processed by fire if it is to enhance our well-being. The most delicious, healthy food we can eat nourishes us only after it has been processed by the fire of digestion. Food that is not well-digested leaves a residue in our system that impedes the functions of our body and so contributes to poor health.

Many thoughts, emotions, and experiences pass through us in the course of a day. We must either allow these to pass through us or we need to process them. Any thoughts, emotions and experiences that we hold onto but do not process actually block the flow of our life-energy. Blocking our life-energy diminishes our well-being and stifles our aliveness.

Strong digestive fire is the foundation of our health — mentally, physically and emotionally.

Fire brightens and focuses the mind. Strength of intellect and sharpness of mind come from fire energy, as does the discrimination we need to make the best choices for ourselves.

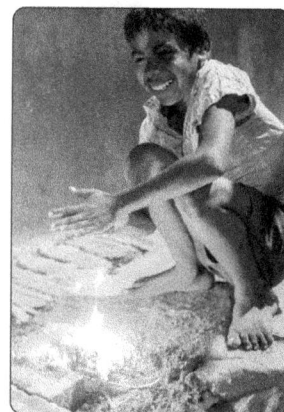

MARTIN JERNBERG | UNSPLASH

Creating our lives and bringing forth our highest potential is a fire process. The *light* of fire illuminates the reality of our circumstances and allows us to see different possibilities; we can then use the *sharpness* of fire to focus our energies and explore those different possibilities; and then, it is through the *transforming* power of fire that something new emerges.

When we have difficulty moving forward with our goals, or if we are feeling unable to take on the tasks and challenges of life, fire can help us to access the drive that we need to get ourselves going. We can *fire ourselves up* by finding an image of fire — contemplating the intensity and transformative power of that fire — and then bringing that fire energy into our body and further stimulating it through a series of Hero poses.

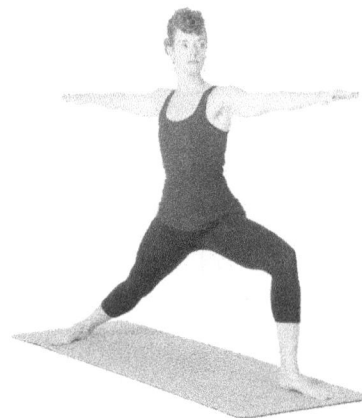

Evoking fire in asana gives our body precision, clarity and vitality. In addition to enhancing our yoga practice, these fire energies help us to safely challenge ourselves in developing strength and flexibility. Heating our body with vigorous asanas melts tension and makes the body more malleable. The focus and heat that we can access through fire allows us to enjoy the challenge of new, advanced and difficult poses.

Fire is related to the **3d chakra**. The seed mantra of the 3rd chakra is *ram*. We can focus on the 3rd chakra and/or chant its seed mantra *ram* in asana, meditation or daily activities to help us balance our fire. (See Appendix on page 227 for more on how to use chakras and seed mantras.)

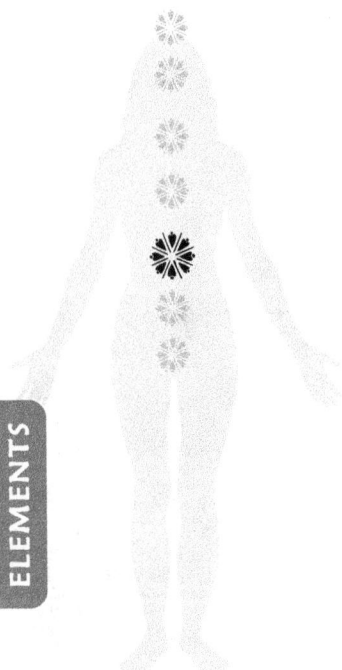

3RD CHAKRA
Element: Fire
Seed mantra: *Ram*

Too Hot or Too Cold

Just as an oven that is too hot burns our food, excess fire in our body damages our tissues and cells. Inflammation, skin rashes, diarrhea and nausea are all expressions of excess fire.

On the emotional level, fire can warm us or damage us depending on how hot the fire is burning. *Balanced fire* gives us emotional warmth to nourish ourselves and our relationships. *Excess fire* creates anger, hatred and irritability which are damaging both to ourselves and the people around us.

On the mental/emotional level, excess heat expresses in *hot-headedness* and *losing our cool*. Our capacity to think well is diminished and the likelihood of our becoming reactive is increased. Without healthy fire our mind and emotions become unbalanced and unclear.

Fire expressing as passion in the heart and mind energizes us creatively. If this passion becomes excessive, however, it *burns us out*.

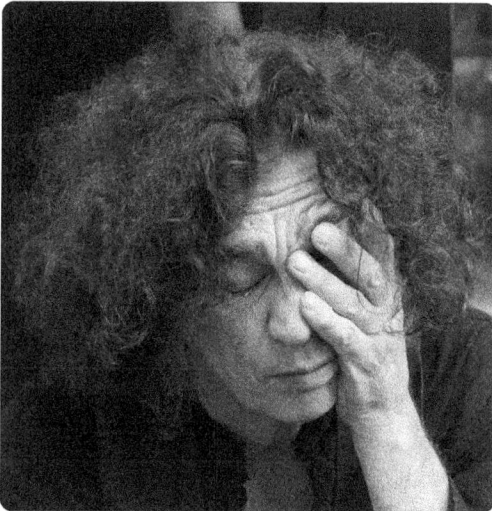

BRUT CARNIOLLUS | UNSPLASH

When our fire is deficient we lose our vitality and our spark. It then becomes difficult to fully engage with life. Fire is our *take-hold* energy. We need fire's energy to whole-heartedly enjoy, fully participate in, and make meaning of life.

Reduce Fire

When our body, mind or emotions are overheated, earth and water are the elemental supports we can engage to cool them down.

Excess fire creates an upward-moving heat in our body, and earth energy helps to draw that heat downward. Connecting to the weight of our body in asana and dropping that weight into the ground, helps us to reduce or prevent the increase of fire. Accessing earth is easiest in reclining poses.

A good basic structure for a fire-balancing asana practice is: Do the asanas using half to three-quarters of your strength-capacity, use long holds, and elongate your exhalations. The hotter your fire is burning, the lower should be the amount of strength-capacity that you use, the gentler should be your holds and the softer should be your elongated exhalations.

Challenging poses, unfamiliar poses and most inversions stimulate fire and so should be avoided if your inner fire is high.

The cooling effect of water is also a natural balance to the heat of excess fire. We can evoke water energy by doing gentle vinyasas together with whole-body breathing. Finding a soft wave-like action in both the vinyasa and the breathing helps to increase their cooling effect.

Elongating the exhalation and shortening the inhalation reduces fire. Working with the breath in this way is most effective when it is done incrementally and sensitively — slightly increasing the length of the exhalation with each breath.

Elongating the exhalation and shortening the inhalation can be used effectively in asana, meditation and in daily life. In asana it can serve as a breath-awareness focus that is integrated throughout a whole practice. Elongated exhalations quiet our body/mind and so enhance meditation. Elongated exhalations together with shortened inhalations can be used as a meditation focus or as a pranayama practice.

An example of using this breathing practice in daily life would be: when walking down a hall at work, count the number of steps you take as you exhale; then add one step at a time to the length of each exhalation until you have reached a comfortable maximum.

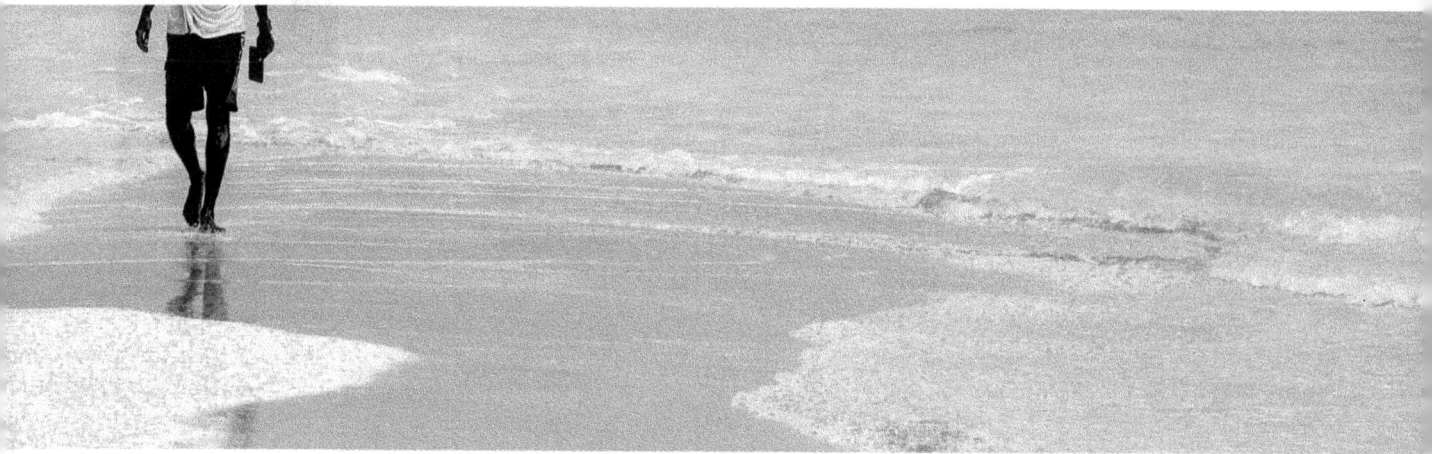

Increase Fire

When our internal fire is low, any vigorous asana practice will stimulate it. Standing poses with strong arm extensions, most inversions and vigorous vinyasas are the most heating.

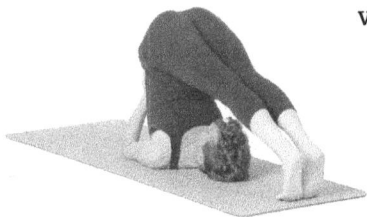

———————————————

Elongating and energizing the spine gives a slight boost to our fire whether we do this in asana or during daily activities.

Heating pranayamas like Bastrika and Kapalabhati* are important fire-building tools, as in lengthening the inhalation and shortening the exhalation. All of these can be put together to create a fire-stimulating pranayama practice.

———————————————

Although not a common practice, I enjoy doing Bastrika and Kapalabhati while holding an asana. I find it both effective and more enjoyable than doing them as seated pranayama.

Meditating on the *very tip* of a candle flame using a sharp, narrow focus helps to increase fire in the mind. This is when we are feeling dull and want to wake ourselves up so we can more fully engage with a task at hand.

*see Appendix, page 228

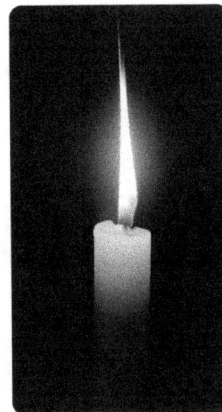

MARC IGNACIO | UNSPLASH

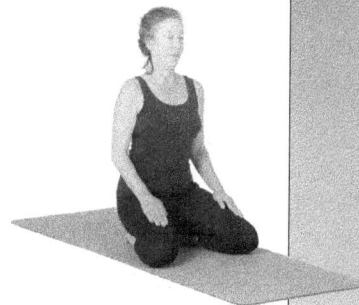

Getting in Touch with Your Inner Fire
🕐 12 - 15 minutes

🔥 Take a **Seated Hero** pose and, if necessary, use a support under your pelvis to make yourself comfortable.

🔥 Take a couple of minutes to let your body/mind settle. Let your pelvis and sitz bones (the bony knobs on the bottom of your pelvis) feel weighted and dropped into the floor.

🔥 Notice the heat in your body. Sense the touch of warm air in your nostrils as you exhale, and sense the relative coolness of the air as you inhale.

🔥 Sense your whole body
  • Would you say that your inner heat is weak or strong?
  • Are you comfortable with the amount of your internal heat as it is in the moment?
  • Are there any parts of your body that feel warmer or cooler than others?

🔥 Move into **Downward Facing Dog**. Hold the position for 1 - 3 minutes. Notice changes in your inner heat during the pose.
  • Does the heat in your body increase?
  • Does heat increase in some parts of your body more than others? Maybe in the head, arms and shoulders?
  • Do you enjoy the sensation of increased heat?

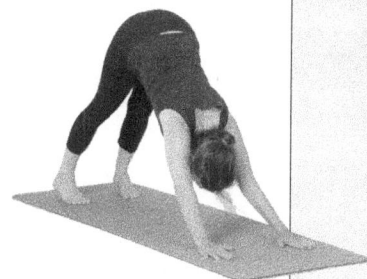

🔥 Return to **Seated Hero**
  • How does your inner heat redistribute through your body as you spend time in Seated Hero?
  • Can you help guide how that heat redistributes? Maybe you can move heat from your chest down to your belly? Or maybe even your pelvis?
  • Trust your capacity to sense and move heat around your body.

🔥 Repeat this process once or twice.

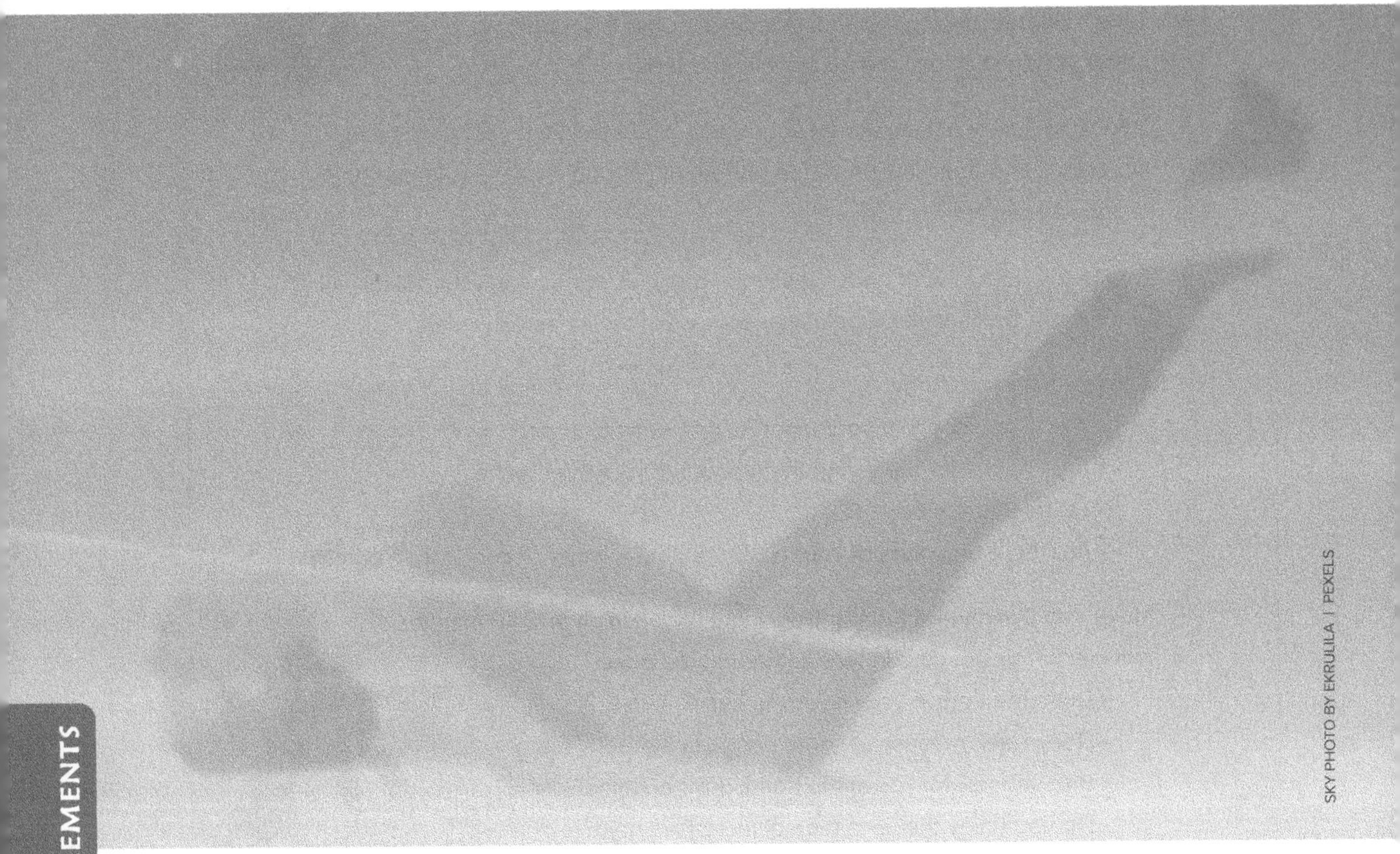

ELEMENTS

SKY PHOTO BY EKRULILA | PEXELS

May our souls
Stay in rhythm
With eternal Breath.
— John O'Donahue

The Elements - Air

Life is movement and air is the elemental source of that movement. All of the movement in our body arises out of the air element.

This is true on every level, from the micro-movements in our cells to our whole body moving through space. Even the movement of thoughts, feelings and emotions are expressions of air.

In exploring air, it is important to remember that we are not talking about the air that we breathe, but rather the primordial air element out of which the air that we breathe arises.

Air is the underlying energy of the physiological functions that keep us alive. Our inner air is the intricate, elegant and miraculous movement of life that is happening in every cell, tissue and organ of our body in every moment of our lives.

When it is balanced, air gives us enthusiasm, playfulness and exuberance. When air is out of balance it throws our life-functions out of balance. From an Ayurvedic perspective, disturbed air is the primary instigator of health problems.

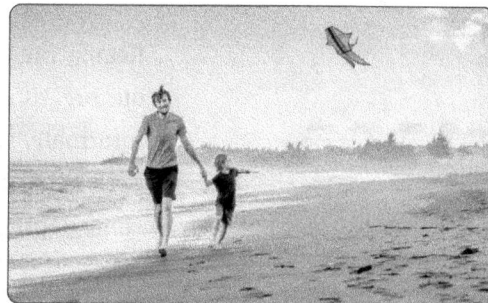

Skillfully managing our air is essential for creating health and well-being. Managing our air means regulating the movement of our body, the movement of our mind/emotions and the movement of our breathing. Yoga practice is designed to do this: asana practice regulates the movement of our body, meditation regulates the mind/emotions, and pranayama regulates the breath.

Air is Unstable

Air is the most unstable of the elements. Air has no inherent restriction on how or where it can move, and its movement can change in a moment. Think about how suddenly that completely still air can turn into a breeze. Equally suddenly a breeze can become a wind, and a wind can turn into a blustery storm. Then as quickly as it began to move, air again can become still.

Air's instability is intimately related to its potency. The interweaving layers of movement in our body that are keeping us alive are able to exist because air's instability allows it to express itself simultaneously in a variety of dynamics of movement, and then quickly change these dynamics according to our body's needs.

The downside of air's instability is that it is prone to going out of balance, which makes air the most difficult element to manage. When our air is balanced, life is good. When air is a little out of balance, life it *less* good. When air is strongly out of balance, it has far-reaching negative effects on our life and well-being.

Breathing and moving are our most immediate needs, and both of these are expressions of the air element. The interrelationship between elemental air, movement and breathing, makes working with the breath one of the most potent aspects of yoga practice.

Regulating our breathing keeps our internal air in balance. We can regulate our breath in asana, pranayama and meditation practice. We can also work informally with breath in daily life. A way of working with breath awareness to balance the air element through our whole body is described in some depth in the upcoming chapter on Prana (see page 121).

Air is related to the **4th chakra** (heart center). *Yam* is the seed mantra of the 4th chakra. The 4th chakra and its mantra *yam* can be used separately or together to add an air-balancing boost to asana. They can also be used together to create a deeply soothing meditation. (See Appendix on page 227 for more on how to use chakras and seed mantras.)

4TH CHAKRA

Element: Air
Seed mantra: *Yam*

Disturbed Air

Air can be a little or a lot disturbed. When it is a lot disturbed it becomes *pushy*. Pushy air does exactly that, it pushes. It pushes other parts of ourselves into disturbance. It *pushes* our thoughts and emotions, it *pushes* the structures and functions of our body, and it *pushes the other elements.*

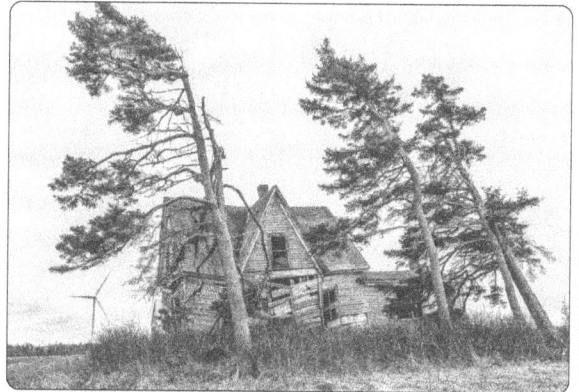

HARRISON HAINES | PEXELS

This dynamic of *air pushing* is important to understand since it is central to Ayurvedic thinking and to how most of our health problems are created. Air is the only element that moves and as such it is an instigator. When air is disturbed it can create problems anywhere in the body.

American's cultural value of achievement and *pushing forward* makes us prone to air disturbances. Highly stimulated air can lead to remarkable creativity and great achievement, but it can also be powerfully destructive. Multi-tasking and pushing ourselves to move faster and go farther than we reasonably can, are related to disturbed air.

Air is light, clear, subtle and mobile. We can experience an air balance or disturbance in any of these qualities on any level: mental, physical or emotional. If one quality is noticeably disturbed the others are likely disturbed or poised to become so.

When our air is balanced, these qualities give us, respectively, light-heartedness, mental clarity, sensitivity and ease of movement. When our air is disturbed, we can recognize that disturbance through an excess in one or more of its qualities.

When we have too much *lightness*, we are ungrounded and unstable. We lose our connection to earth. Excessive amounts of *clarity* and *subtlety* make us hypersensitive. Ordinary life challenges that roll off our backs when we are in balance become intolerable when air's clear and subtle qualities are aggravated.

When the *mobile* quality of air is aggravated, it expresses in us as movement that is erratic, unstable and agitated. It is as if we are being blown around by a capricious wind.

Air is the only element that moves and as such it is an instigator. When air is disturbed it can create problems anywhere in the body.

Balance Air

We must use our air skillfully or it can become the servant that takes control of the house. Imbalanced air moves excessively and erratically. Our first step in pacifying disturbed air is breaking its momentum by slowing ourselves down or stopping. Stopping and settling, for even a few minutes puts a brake on disturbed air.

Regulating our breath is the most direct way of keeping our air balanced. One of the simplest and most effective ways of using our breathing to balance our air is to lengthen the exhalation and shorten the inhalation. This is an important practice because when our air is disturbed we are almost certainly breathing with a dominant inhalation and incomplete exhalation.

In lengthening the exhalation and shortening the inhalation, sensitively encouraging the breath is more effective than trying to control it. We can explore this breath pattern as part of a pranayama practice or integrate it in asana practice. Periodically touching into this way of breathing throughout our day helps keep our air balanced.

Another pleasant and effective way of using the breath to balance air is inhaling as if we are breathing in directly through the heart, then exhaling down through the legs and into the ground. This practice, too, lends itself well to us using it throughout the day to keep ourselves balanced.

Earth is our best elemental resource for balancing disturbed air. Tuning into the weight and solidity of our body gives us access to earth energy. Restorative and reclining asana are the go-to practices for awakening our earth.

It is always helpful to remember that our body is made of earth and that we need only to slow down in order to connect to its support.

Breath Awareness

🕐 7 - 12 minutes

Lie on your back with a small folded towel supporting the back of your lungs and heart.

🌀 Take time to let yourself settle into this position, adjusting the towel for comfort if needed. Notice how the towel supports the lungs and encourages the chest to open.

🌀 Become aware of the sensation of the movement of your breathing.

🌀 Imagine that you are inside the center of your lungs — from this perspective be aware of the three-dimensional movement of your lungs as you breathe. Continue for 2 - 3 minutes.

🌀 Let go of any ideas of how the breath should be moving. However you are breathing is fine. Pretending that you are half-asleep helps you to let go of the tendency to control the breath and so your natural breathing can more easily express.

🌀 Rest for a few breaths.

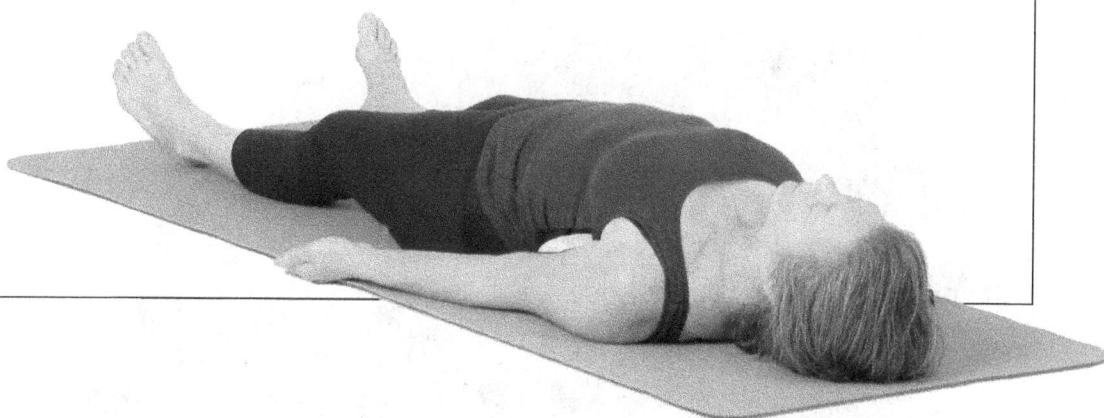

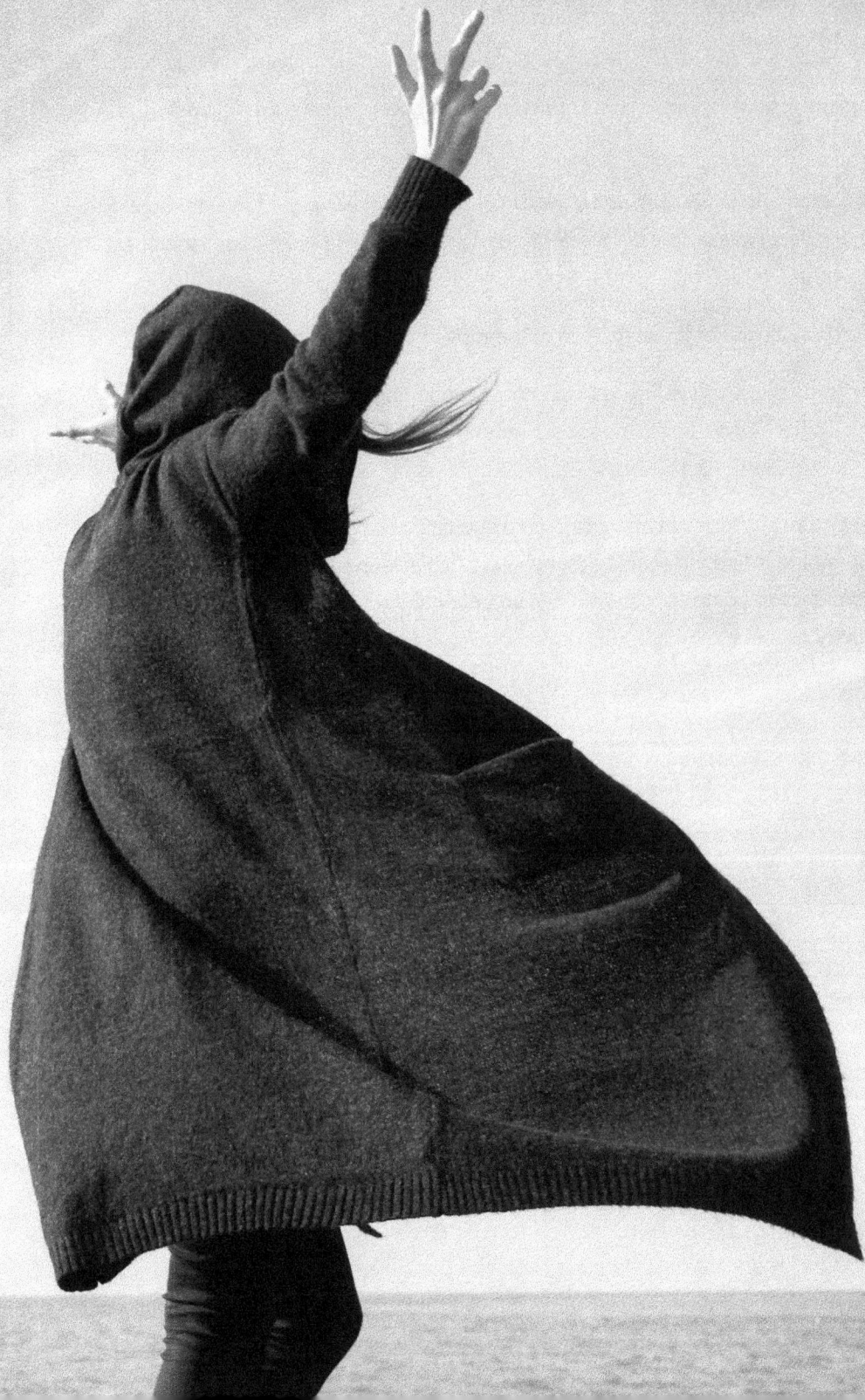

EXPLORING AIR

Breathing and Moving 🕑 7 - 12 minutes

🌀 Bend your knees and place your feet flat on the floor.

🌀 Return to the awareness of your breathing, imagining that you are inside the center of your lungs with awareness of their three-dimensional movement.

🌀 Expand that awareness to include the movement of your ribcage as you breathe. Continue for 2 - 3 minutes.

🌀 With very small, easy movements, begin alternating between arching your lower back away from the floor and pressing it into the floor. Keep your spine and pelvis relaxed, allowing them to respond to the movement of your breath/lower back movement. What is most important is that the movement is easy and natural.

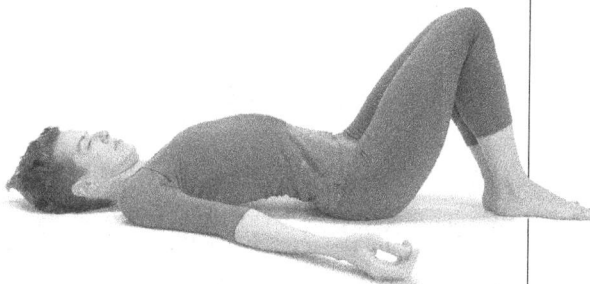

🌀 Let the arching of your lower back away from the floor merge with your inhalation, and let the pressing of your lower back into the floor merge with the exhalation.

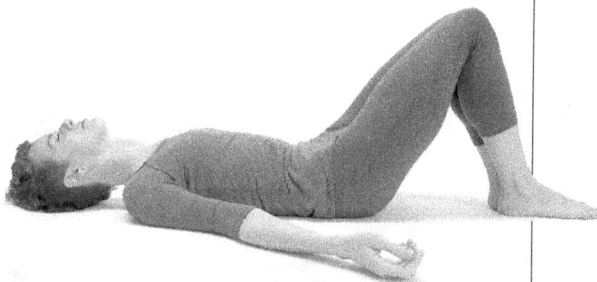

Small, soft movements allow the lower back and breathing to feel as if they belong together. The movement quality that you are cultivating is similar to floating in water and allowing your breath and lower back to be moved by gentle waves. There is a feeling that you are being moved and breathed, rather than you doing the moving and breathing.

🌀 As you yield into this body/breath movement, notice how the rest of your body begins subtly to respond to this movement. Stay with this until you have a sense that the movement is so natural that it would continue if you fell asleep.

🌀 Rest briefly.

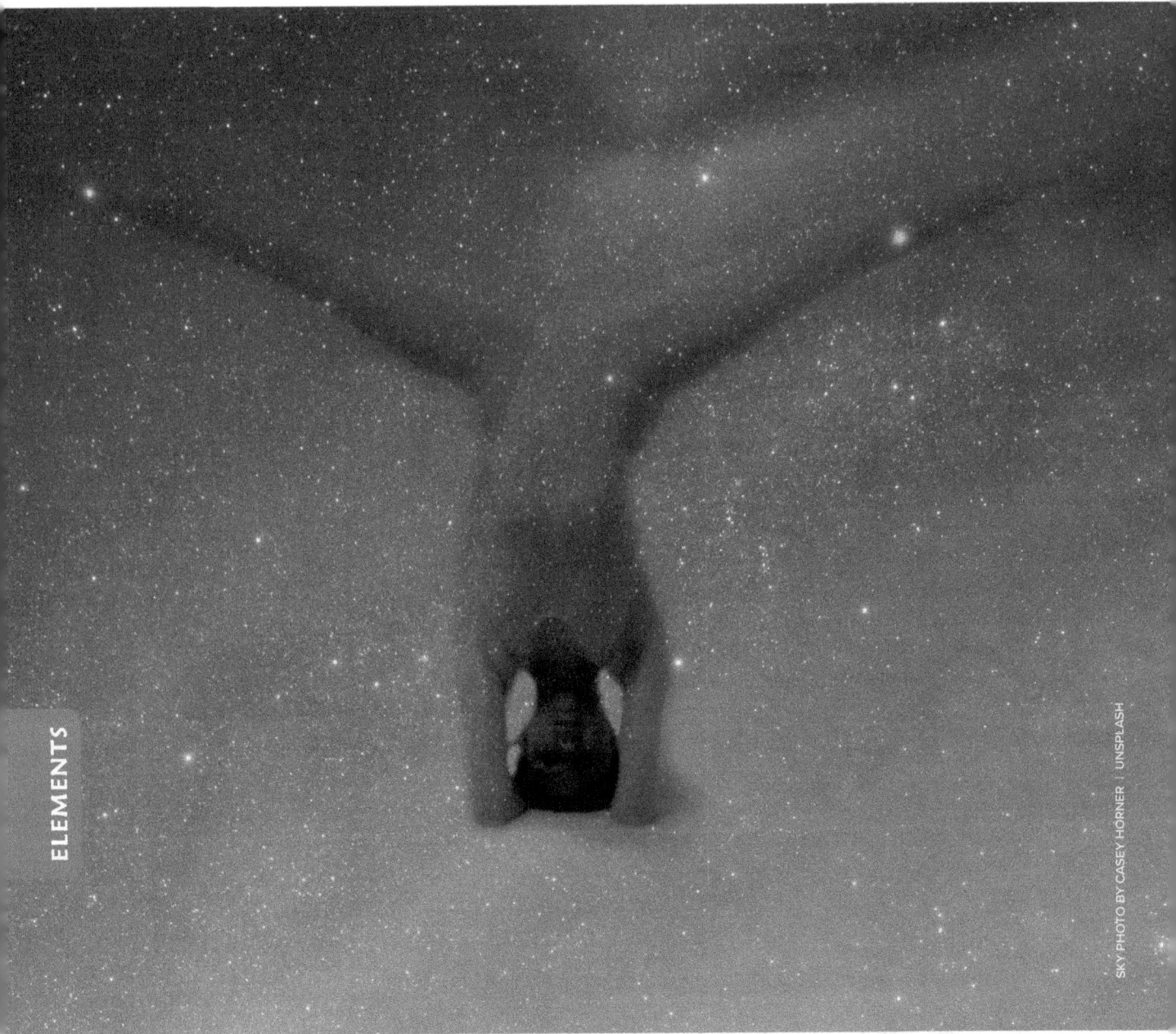

ELEMENTS

SKY PHOTO BY CASEY HORNER | UNSPLASH

Space is love.

— *Dr. Vasant Lad*

The Elements - Space

Space makes all things possible. It is the field in which life happens.

Space has no palpable substance, heat or movement of its own but it is through space that the substance, heat and movement of the other elements exist and can be felt. Everything inside of our body and in the external world is suspended in and supported by space.

Space is in the background of our awareness. We take it for granted. Bringing space into the foreground of our awareness lets us see things in a different light, which opens us to new perspectives and new possibilities. Awareness of space enriches us by giving us an added perceptual dimension. Our relationship to ourselves, to others and to the experiences of life is different when we include space in our awareness.

We express our intuitive understanding of the importance of space with phrases as such "expanding the mind," "opening the heart" and "connecting to our larger selves." Most of us know the discomfort of acting with a closed mind or a closed heart. Relationships are often a dance around spatial needs, with some people wanting less space and others wanting more.

Wisdom, love and compassion are three of the most important life-enhancing capacities that we can cultivate. All of these require increased inner spaciousness. All of these require a greater capacity to be inclusive of people, new ideas and all of the variables of life. Wisdom, love and compassion require us to *open* our minds and hearts.

A deeply imprinted memory from my Ayurvedic training was Dr. Lad masterfully guiding us in a meditation that step-by-step took us to an experience that *space is love*. I wish I could describe the process but sadly I cannot remember it. I still, however, have a visceral memory of

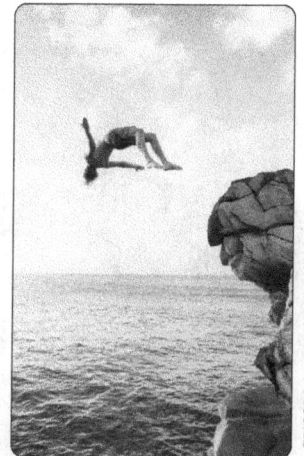

EPICSTOCK | DREAMSTIME

my experience of space being love, and my utter surprise of how obvious it seemed. I also remember Dr. Lad's last sentence, *"there can be no love without space."*

As an example, when we are challenged in a yoga practice we tend to concentrate harder to meet that challenge. In this increased concentration we often narrow our focus in a way that tightens our body and so we end up working against ourselves. We are likely to have more success in dealing with a challenge if we can hold a clear focus while staying connected to the space around our body. If indeed space is love, then when we open space around our challenge, we are surrounding it in love which automatically makes the challenge less difficult.

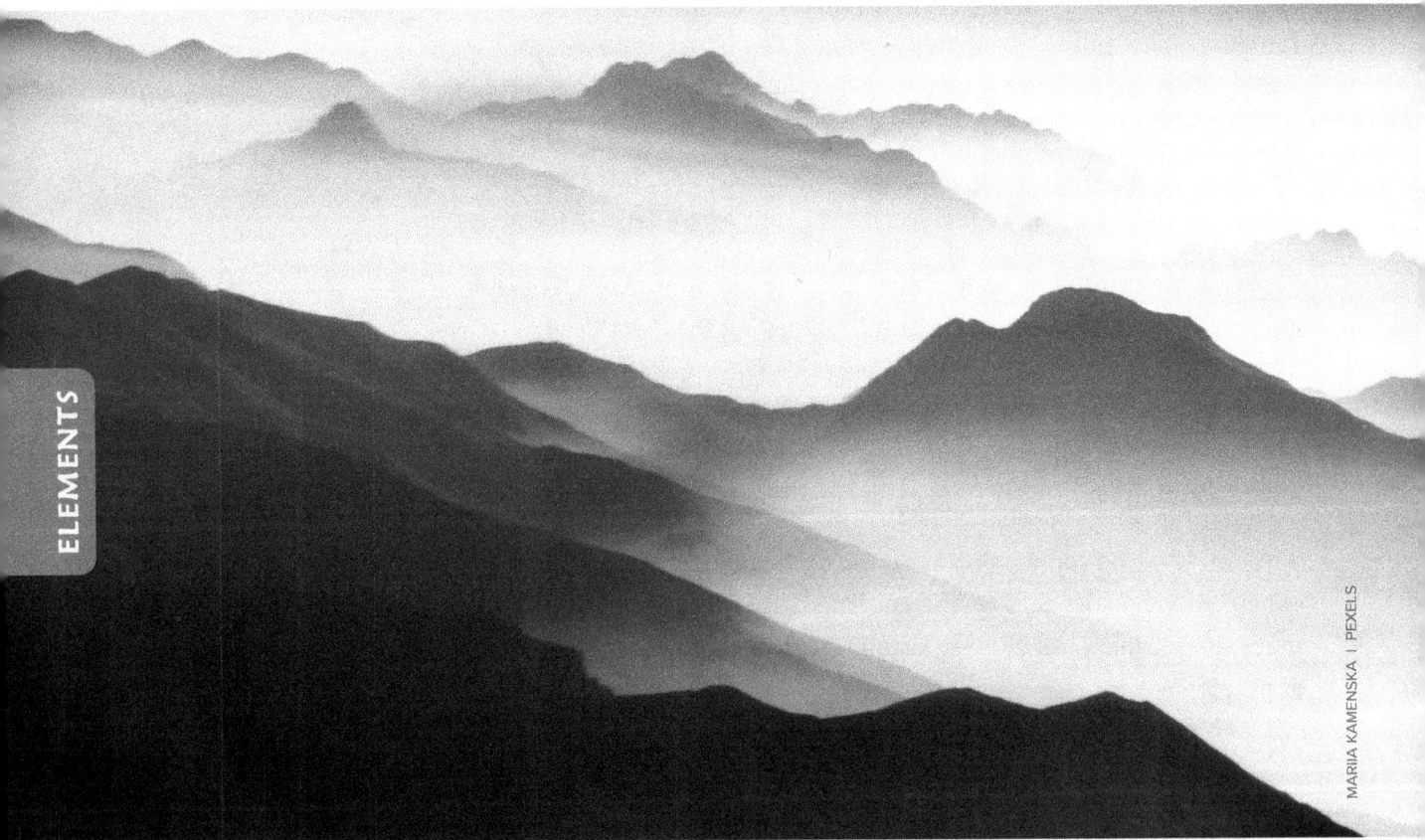

ELEMENTS

MARIIA KAMENSKA | PEXELS

Exploring different sizes of space in different situations is how we discover what helps us the most. We can use any amount of space from an inch or so around the body up to the size of the room we are in. In meditation or in a meditative approach to asana and pranayama we can even explore opening our awareness to the end of the universe.

───────────────

On a more concrete level, including the awareness of space in our yoga practice tends to give us greater ease and increased strength. This happens because our body works in a more integrated way when we are connected to the space around us. The larger perspective that we get from space also allows for new insights into refining our practice and working more skillfully with ourselves when facing our limitations.

Our needs for space are fluid, and they are different for different people. On any given day our needs for space change depending on our mental and emotional state. If we are sad, we well might want to go to bed or curl up in a corner. Smaller spaces tend to be more comforting when we are feeling vulnerable. If we are in a saddened state, meditation, pranayama and reclining asanas are akin to smaller space and so are more comforting than expansive asanas.

On the other hand, when we are feeling confident and open, a small space is confining and does not allow us to fully express ourselves. This is the time for expansive asana and challenging ourselves with new practices.

Trusting ourselves and treating ourselves kindly is essentially giving ourselves the space to be who we are. We want to keep our internal space as free as possible from judging thoughts or negative feelings. Every living thing is happier and healthier when it has the space to be itself. Giving the people in our lives the space to be who they are fosters nourishing relationships. Establishing the intention to give ourselves the space to be who we are is a perfect way to enter a yoga practice.

On any given day our needs for space change depending on our mental and emotional state.

───────────────

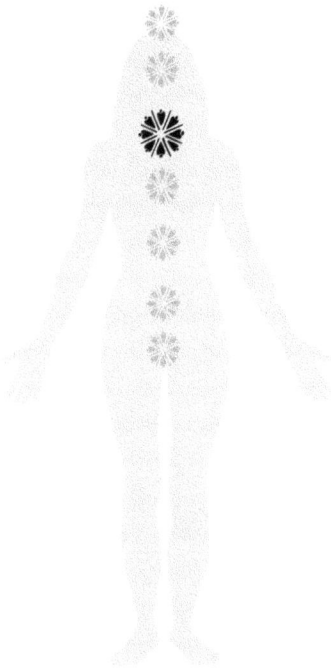

Space is related to the **5th chakra**. *Hum* is the seed mantra of the 5th chakra. Space and its seed mantra can be used individually or together for clearing, opening and connecting to our internal or external space. (See Appendix on page 227 for more on how to use chakras and seed mantras.)

Too Much or Too Little Space

Musculoskeletal pain is often caused by compression, and compression is essentially a lack of space. For example, the tiniest bit of compression on a nerve root can create tremendous pain while the tiniest increase of space around a nerve root can relieve pain. Creating space both inside an area of pain and around it can relieve pain, sometimes dramatically.

Tension and poor posture are two common causes of compression in our body. Poor posture and tension go hand-in-hand so by improving our posture we gain the structural support that we need to let go of tension.

The reduced internal space created by compression and tension can create other problems for us. Blood and nerve flow to cells, tissues and organs are reduced and so our physiological health is compromised. Too little space in our body also makes us stiff and uncoordinated, which inclines

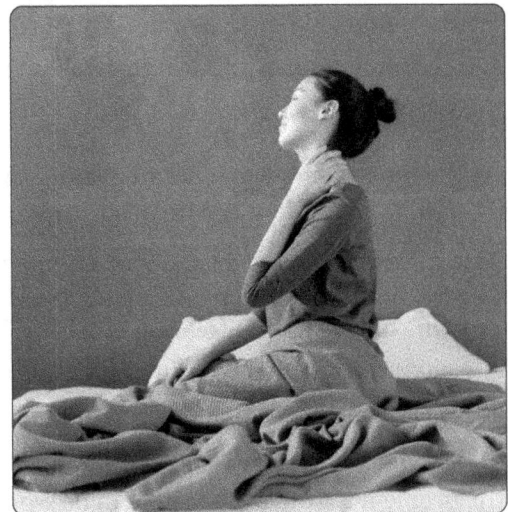

5TH CHAKRA

Element: Space
Seed mantra: *Hum*

ELEMENTS

us toward using excess effort in whatever we do — including asanas. We can focus on opening internal space through stretching, breathing and imagery. We can also create more internal space by reaching through the periphery of our body.

When we have too little mental/emotional space, our thinking narrows and our feelings become constricted. Without inner spaciousness, our thoughts and emotions can become intense, compressed and unmanageable. When we feel caught in restrictive mental and emotional patterns, creating even a little space around them can give us relief. Meditation is our friend for accessing more mental and emotional space.

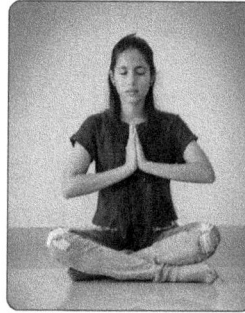

PRANAV KUMAR JAIN | UNSPLASH

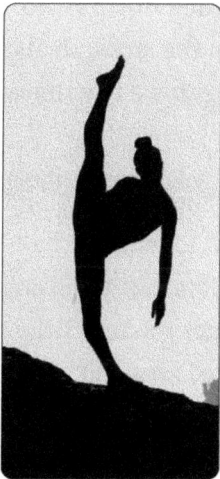

DAVID HOFMANN | UNSPLASH

Physically, too much space in the body is related to physical instability and hypermobility. Hypermobile people are frequently looked at with envy because of how easily they seem to do advanced poses. A hyper-mobile body, however, is prone to having mysterious pain and to being easily injured. The instability of their bodies and their vulnerability to injury makes it challenging for these people to develop strength.

Hypermobility can also be related to health problems including anxiety, autoimmune issues, insomnia and poor digestion.*

It is important for people with hypermobile joints to maintain joint integrity when doing asanas. Simple asanas done with longer holds that allow time to focus on joint stability is useful for these people.

Spaciousness allows us to be open and generous to ourselves and others. Too much space, however, leaves us spacey, easily disoriented and ungrounded.

*see Appendix, page 230, for more information

Play with Space

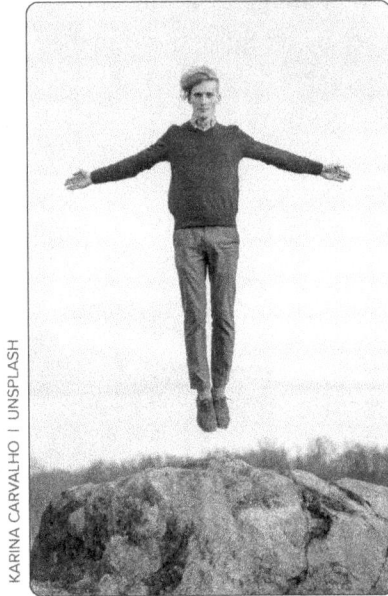

KARINA CARVALHO | UNSPLASH

Being aware of the space around us when doing yoga awakens whole-body awareness. This allows us to see options for refining a practice that are not available when we are using a narrow focus. A narrow focus makes it more likely that we will do a practice using our body in habitual ways rather than being open to discovering new ways.

Connecting to external space during asana gives us a surprising amount of strength and ease. You can experiment with this by: stretching your arms out to the side at shoulder height and notice how it feels. Bring your arms down and take a brief rest. Again, lift your arms to the same position and this time reach your arms and fingers into the space beyond your fingertips. Notice any difference in the strength and ease in your arm and through your whole body. Repeating this a few times can help to clarify the difference.

When we come up against a physical restriction in asana there are a couple of ways that we can use space to help us release it. Extending the periphery of our body into the space around us and simultaneously sensing the restriction as part of whole-body awareness encourages the restriction to yield. We can also focus our breathing into the restricted area and use the inhalation and/or exhalation to create space around and within the restriction.

A different option is to do an asana that puts a subtle pressure into the area of restriction, then place your attention in the center of the restriction and use the exhalation to open a tiny space in that center. Initially the space will be as tiny as the head of a pin — as you stay with the process, the space will become larger and the area of restriction will become more permeable.

ELEMENTS

We can think about **hypermobility** as a lack of spatial integrity. The whole-body integration that happens when we cultivate awareness of the space around our body helps to reduce the tendency of a hypermobile body to collapse into individual joints.

The laxity in the ligaments and tendons of hypermobile joints needs to be balanced by muscular action that increases joint stability. This muscular action can be both whole-body and localized around the joints. Good body alignment is the foundation of balanced whole-body muscular action.

In working with the muscles around the joints an astringent action can be effective. The astringent, puckering action that happens in our mouth when we eat a lemon is a similar to the tonifying action that we want to awaken in the muscles around loose joints.

This tonifying action is created around the entire circumference of the joint, and it is done together with a focus on creating space inside the joint. The astringent, tonifying muscular action is used to sustain the space inside the joint. It is not necessarily easy or obvious as to how to do this, but it is effective and worth exploring as support for working the special challenges of a hypermobile body.

> *"Ayurveda encourages you to be an active participant in your own journey toward healing. This involves learning about your relationship with the elements and the unique combinations they create called doshas."*
>
> *— www.banyanbotanicals.com*

Exploring Internal Space

- Come into **Mountain** pose. Sense/imagine your whole body being empty. Take time to allow this experience to develop.

- Maintain the sense of your body being empty and further develop this internal space while doing the movement sequence on the facing page.

  You can do this as a vinyasa, as individual poses held for a period of time, or as a combination of both. If you do this as a vinyasa, it is easier to explore internal space when the movement is slower.

- Throughout the movement, pause when you notice an area of tension and release that tension by opening space within it.

- Repeat the series once or twice then rest briefly in **Mountain** pose.

Exploring External Space

- In **Mountain** pose, relax your eyes and come into peripheral vision. Become aware of the space around your whole body. Take a few moments to allow this experience to develop.

- Maintain and further develop this awareness of the space around you as you repeat the movement sequence.

- Repeat once or twice then rest briefly in **Mountain** pose.

Exploring Internal and External Space

- In **Mountain** pose let the skin on your whole body soften to allow your internal space to merge with the external space. Take a few moments to allow this experience to develop.

- Maintain and further develop this sense of merged internal and external space as you repeat the movement sequence two or three times.

- Rest in **Savasana** as long as you like.

ELEMENTS

Mountain Pose with Forward Bend 🕐 12 - 18 minutes

Each of the explorations on the facing page uses this same series of poses.

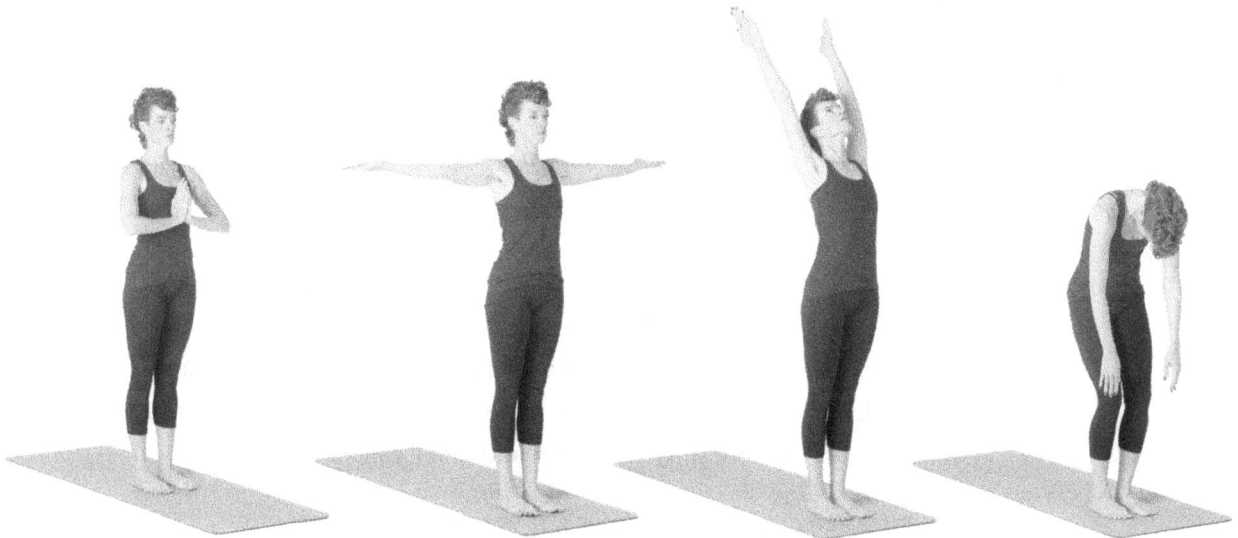

Come into **Mountain** pose

Open your arms to the side, then extend them...

...over your head, coming into a slight **Backbend.**

Fold forward...

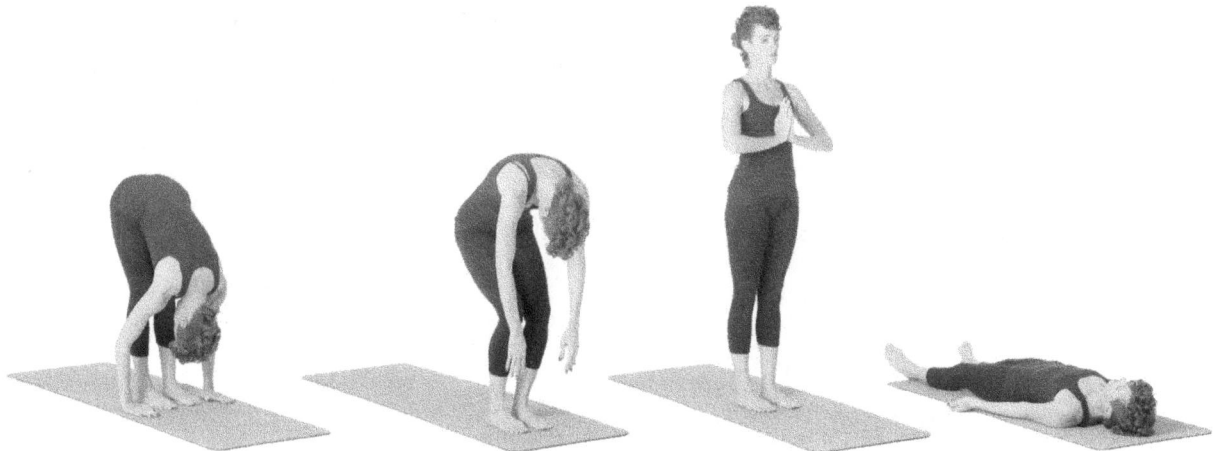

...into **Forward Bend**...

...then roll up through your spine to come back to...

...**Mountain** pose.

Rest in **Savasana** after the three explorations.

Speaking of Space

Our most obvious relationship to external space when doing yoga is with our practice space. If we enjoy our practice space we are more likely to go there. It can be insightful to sit in your practice space and ask yourself how welcoming it feels to you. Are there any adjustments that you can make to it so it more fully welcomes and inspires you?

An uncluttered space with a touch of beauty like a flower or candle is welcoming. Candles and flowers hint of ritual and so invite us to open to new possibilities. A statue, photograph, something from nature or any personal object that holds meaning for us can gather our energies and inspire us. Having a couple of practice-related books close by gives us easy access to information and inspiration.

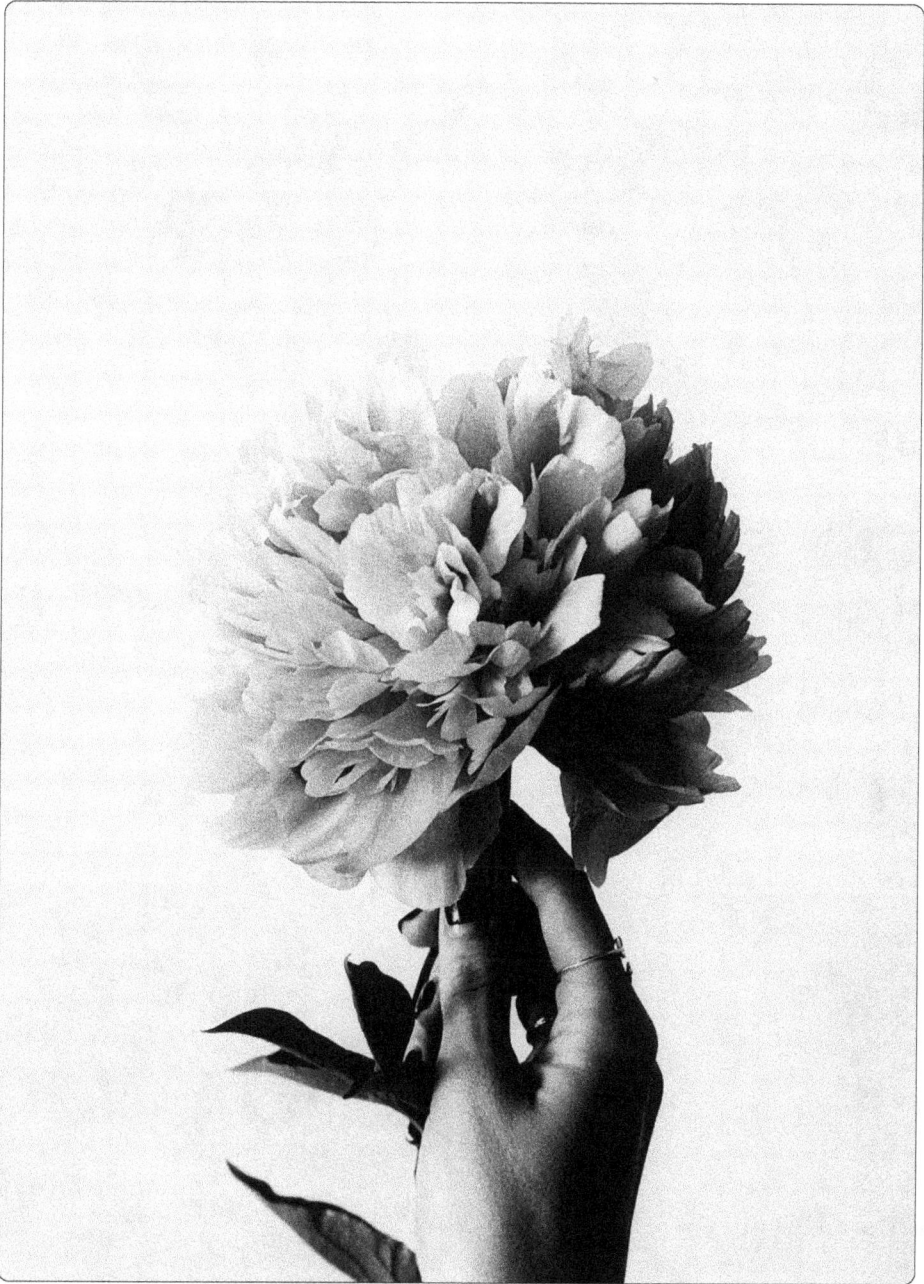

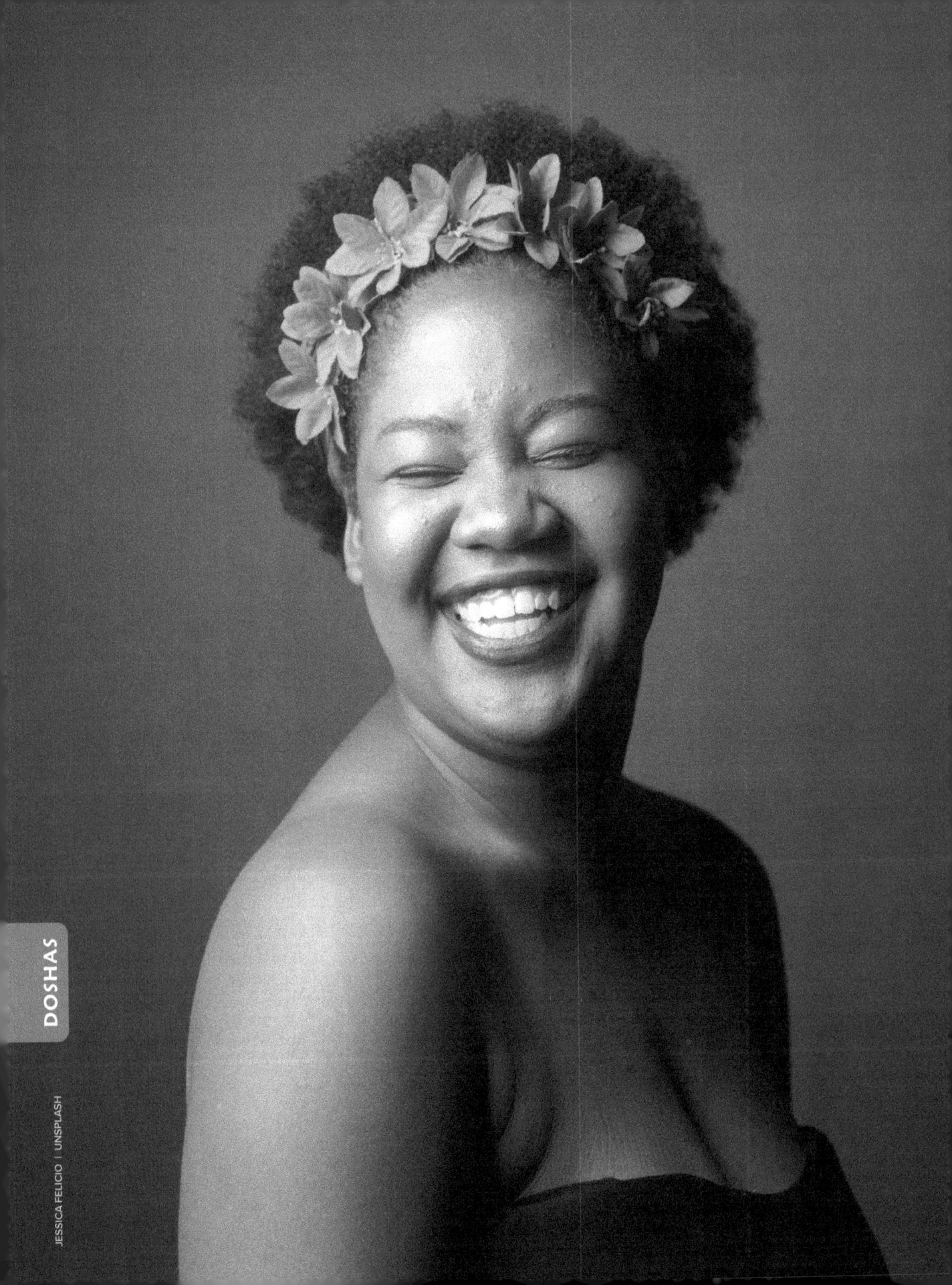

What Are the Doshas?

At the center of Ayurveda's approach to creating health is its signature principle — the doshas. Doshas are a way of looking at the underlying energy/matter of health and happiness. Working with the doshas is working with this underlying energy/matter.

Having *balanced doshas* is Ayurveda's way of saying that we are healthy; physically, mentally and emotionally. Balancing our doshas means balancing ourselves. Health and happiness are the goals of Ayurveda, and *balancing our doshas* is the Ayurvedic means of reaching these goals.

Our goal in applying Ayurveda to yoga is to balance the doshas.

The doshas describe how the Five Elements function in our body. There are three doshas and each dosha is a combination of two elements. Our discussion and explorations of the Five Elements in the last section gave us the foundation for understanding the doshas and their *personalities*.

VATA is made up of air and space. Air is the underlying energy of the movement in our body and space is the container in which air moves.

PITTA is a combination of fire and water. Fire is the dominant energy in pitta. Water simply helps to spread and temper the heat of pitta's fire.

KAPHA is a combination of earth and water. Earth is the dominant energy in kapha but water plays a major role in all the functions of the body.

THE DOSHAS AND THEIR ELEMENTS

VATA
- Air + Space

PITTA
- Fire + Water

KAPHA
- Earth + Water

Everyone has all three doshas, but in different quantities. If we have a predominance of vata dosha, we are said to have a vata constitution. A predominance of pitta dosha gives us a pitta constitution, and a predominance of kapha dosha gives us a kapha constitution. Less commonly, people can have equal amounts of two doshas, and even less commonly, equal amounts of all three doshas.

Our doshic constitution was set in place at conception and remains the reference for health throughout our life.

Every part of our body is made up of all three doshas with different areas of the body having a greater or lesser amount of individual doshas. In addition, each dosha has an area of the torso in which it dominates. This area is referred to as the dosha's *home site*. A doshic imbalance originates in the dosha's home site, and so these sites are among the most important areas of focus when using yoga practice to balance doshas.

In this section you will discover how the doshas express themselves as *living* principles in our body, mind and emotions. You will learn how to recognize doshic disturbances in their early stages, together with on-the-go interventions for antidoting those disturbances.

DOSHIC HOME SITES

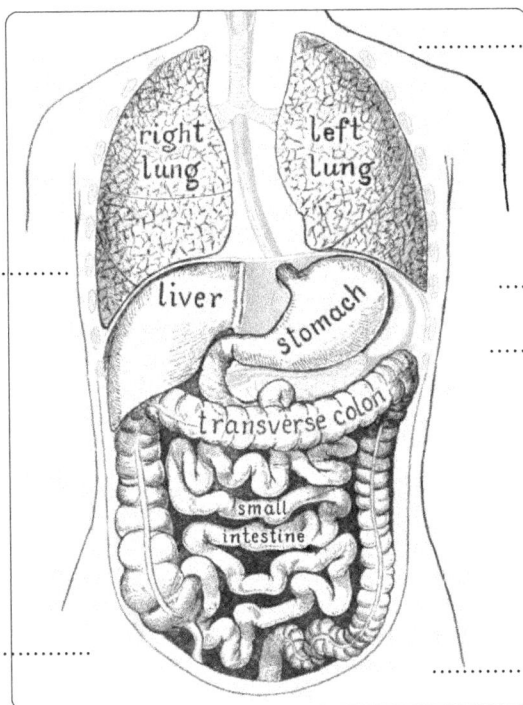

KAPHA
• LUNGS

PITTA
• STOMACH
• LIVER
• SMALL INTESTINE

VATA
• COLON

DR. JOHANNES SOBOTTA, SOBOTTA'S ATLAS & TEXT-BOOK OF HUMAN ANATOMY 1906 | WIKIMEDIA COMMONS

DOSHAS

Entering Our Doshic World

Being alive means that we are in constant flux. We are always changing, sometimes in small ways and sometimes in large ones. This makes life interesting and it allows us to learn and to grow.

The doshas are living processes in our body and so they, too, are in constant flux.

Being in constant flux means that we are unstable. We are always shifting into and out of balance. When this shifting is subtle we are expressing the natural rhythm of health. We are maintaining equilibrium. If our going in and out of balance happens in large swings or if we get stuck in an imbalance, then we have lost our equilibrium and our well-being is diminished. An example of a large swing is when we work intensively for a period of time and then collapse or get sick.

The ongoing dance between balance and imbalance happens in all aspects of our life. Hunger is a message that we are subtly out of balance and that we need food in order to regain balance. If we eat when we are hungry we sustain our equilibrium. If we do not eat reasonably soon after recognizing hunger, our imbalance strengthens and we may experience nausea, irritability or impaired thinking.

A version of this scenario happens in all of the many imbalance/balance cycles that occur every day of our lives. All of our needs are cyclical including our need for water, exercise, sleep, activity, work, medications, community, solitude, etc. We need the right amount of these to stay balanced. Too much or too little throws us off balance. Our well-being depends mightily on how we navigate the natural balance/imbalance cycles of our life.

Our well-being depends mightily on how we navigate the natural balance/imbalance cycles of our life.

In those inevitable times when we become ill, we can use our understanding of doshic balancing and yoga to give concentrated support to our body to help it regain health.

Prakriti and Vrikriti

Prakriti
is our doshic
constitution.

Vrikriti
is a doshic
disturbance.

We do not need to learn a lot of Sanskrit terms in order to use Ayurveda for enhancing yoga practice. A few terms, however, are helpful to know because they express concepts that are lacking in English. *Prakriti* and *vrikriti* are two of these. Prakriti is our doshic constitution, and vrikriti is a doshic disturbance.

As previously mentioned, most of us are predominantly one dosha and that dosha determines our *doshic constitution* or *prakriti*. It is possible to have equal amounts of two doshas or all three doshas. In these cases we would have respectively a bi-doshic or tri-doshic constitution. Prakriti is our personal configuration of doshas.

Prakriti is set in place at conception and remains throughout our life. Like our DNA, our prakriti contains the seeds of who we are. It determines our strengths, weaknesses and tendencies. It is the underlying blueprint around which our body, mind and personality develop. Prakriti is our life-long reference for maintaining health.

Out-of-balance doshas are referred to as a *vrikriti*. A vrikriti tells us which of our doshas are disturbed, the nature of that disturbance and in what part of the body the disturbance is happening. Vrikriti is the information that Ayurveda uses to determine what is needed to regain doshic balance. We can be imbalanced in any dosha but are more likely to go out of balance in our dominant dosha.

Doshas Have Homes — Home Sites

Every cell, tissue and organ in our body is composed of all three doshas. Different areas of our body, however, have lesser or greater amounts of specific doshic activity. The most significant of these areas of doshic dominance are in the vital organs. Each dosha has an area in the vital organs where it has a home site. It is in its *home site* that a doshic disturbance begins.

The home site of vata is in the colon. The home site of pitta is the stomach, liver and small intestine. The home site of kapha is the lungs.

Tuning into these areas is a way of developing sensitivity to the beginning of a doshic disturbance. Being aware of a doshic disturbance when it is just starting allows us to re-balance it quickly and so prevent it from becoming stronger and potentially more problematic. It is easy to balance a doshic disturbance in its early stage and increasingly difficult as the disturbance becomes more established.

How Do I Know My Doshic Nature

Having a consultation with an Ayurvedic doctor or practitioner is the most reliable way to find out your prakriti. Many self-tests are available to help people explore their doshic nature. You will gain much understanding of Ayurveda and of yourself through self-tests. Self-testing will also help you learn how to think about yourself from an Ayurvedic perspective. See page 94 for the test.

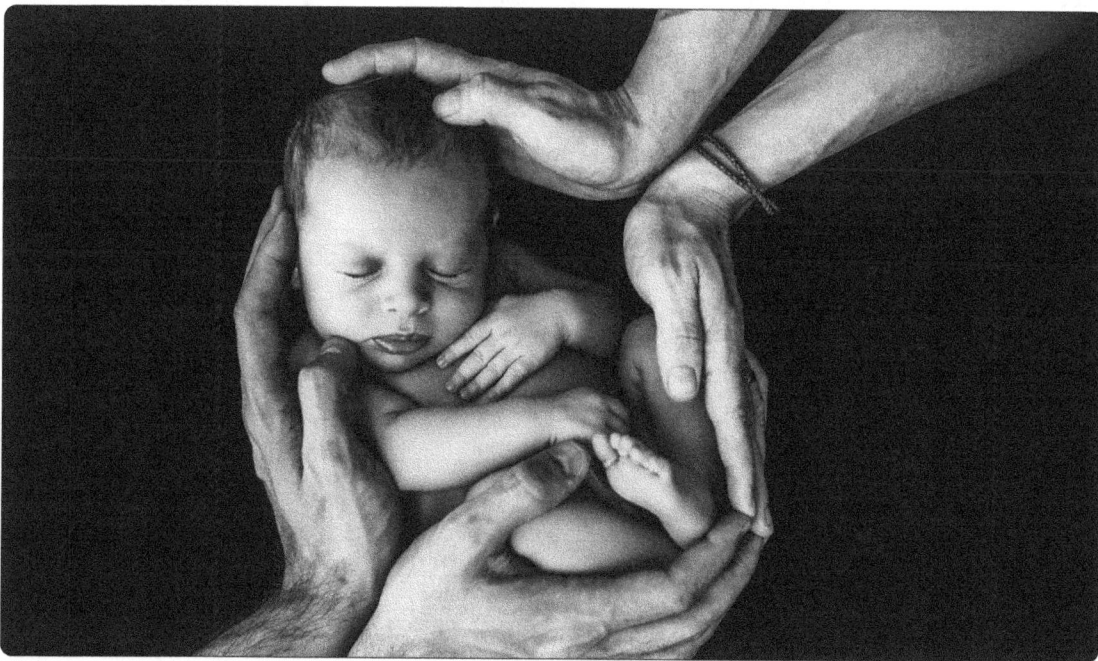

ISAAC QUESADA | UNSPLASH

Guidelines for Determining Your Constitution

Enjoy the following self-test that was generously provided by the Ayurvedic Institute:

To determine your constitution it is best to fill out the chart twice. First, base your choices on what is most consistent over a long period of your life (your prakruti). Then, fill out a second chart, responding to how you have been feeling more recently (your vikruti).

PRAKRITI

	VATA	PITTA	KAPHA
BODY SIZE	Slim	Medium	Large
BODY WEIGHT	Low	Medium	Overweight
CHIN	Thin, angular	Tapering	Rounded, double
CHEEKS	Wrinkled, sunken	Smooth, flat	Rounded, plump
EYES	Small, sunken, dry, active, black, brown, nervous	Sharp, bright, gray, green, yellow/red, sensitive to light	Big, beautiful, blue, calm, loving
NOSE	Uneven shape, deviated septum	Long pointed, red nose-tip	Short rounded, button nose
LIPS	Dry, cracked, black/brown tinge	Red, inflamed, yellowish	Smooth, oily, pale, whitish
TEETH	Stick out, big, roomy, thin gums	Medium, soft, tender gums	Healthy, white, strong gums
SKIN	Thin, dry, cold, rough, dark	Smooth, oily, warm, rosy	Thick, oily, cool, white, pale
HAIR	Dry, brown, black, knotted brittle, scarce	Straight, oily, blond, gray, red, bald	Thick, curly, oily, wavy, luxuriant
NAILS	Dry, rough, brittle, break easily	Sharp, flexible, pink, lustrous	Thick, oily, smooth, polished
NECK	Thin, tall	Medium	Big, folded
CHEST	Flat, sunken	Moderate	Expanded, round
BELLY	Thin, flat, sunken	Moderate	Big, pot-bellied
BELLY BUTTON	Small, irregular, herniated	Oval, superficial	Big, deep, round, stretched
HIPS	Slender, thin	Moderate	Heavy, big
JOINTS	Cold, cracking	Moderate	Large, lubricated
APPETITE	Irregular, scanty	Strong, unbearable	Slow but steady
DIGESTION	Irregular, forms gas	Quick, causes burning	Prolonged, forms mucous
TASTE	Sweet, sour, salty	Sweet, bitter, astringent	Bitter, pungent, astringent
THIRST	Changeable	Surplus	Sparse
ELIMINATION	Constipation	Loose	Thick, oily, sluggish
Physical ACTIVITY	Hyperactive	Moderate	Slow
Mental ACTIVITY	Hyperactive	Moderate	Dull, slow
EMOTIONS	Anxiety, fear, uncertainty	Anger, hate, jealousy	Calm, greedy, attachment
FAITH	Variable	Extremist	Consistent
INTELLECT	Quick but faulty response	Accurate response	Slow, exact
RECOLLECTION	Recent good, remote poor	Distinct	Slow and sustained
DREAMS	Quick, active, many, fearful	Fiery, war, violence	Lakes, snow, romantic
SLEEP	Scanty, broken up, sleeplessness	Little but sound	Deep, prolonged
SPEECH	Rapid, unclear	Sharp, penetrating	Slow, monotonous
FINANCIAL	Poor, spends on trifles	Spends on luxuries	Rich, good money preserver
TOTALS	VATA	PITTA	KAPHA

DOSHAS

Sometimes it helps to have a friend ask you the questions and fill in the chart for you, as they may have insight (and impartiality) to offer.

After finishing the charts, add up the number of marks in each column. This will help you discover your own ratio of doshas in your prakruti and vikruti. Most people will have one dosha predominant, a few will have two doshas approximately equal and even fewer will have all three doshas in equal proportion. For instance, if your vikruti shows more pitta than your prakruti, you will want to follow a pitta-soothing regimen to try and bring your vikruti back into balance with your prakruti. If your prakruti and vikruti seem about the same, then you would choose the regimen of your strongest dosha.

VRIKRITI   Date:

BODY SIZE	○ Slim	○ Medium	○ Large
BODY WEIGHT	○ Low	○ Medium	○ Overweight
CHIN	○ Thin, angular	○ Tapering	○ Rounded, double
CHEEKS	○ Wrinkled, sunken	○ Smooth, flat	○ Rounded, plump
EYES	○ Small, sunken, dry, active, black, brown, nervous	○ Sharp, bright, gray, green, yellow/red, sensitive to light	○ Big, beautiful, blue, calm, loving
NOSE	○ Uneven shape, deviated septum	○ Long pointed, red nose-tip	○ Short rounded, button nose
LIPS	○ Dry, cracked, black/brown tinge	○ Red, inflamed, yellowish	○ Smooth, oily, pale, whitish
TEETH	○ Stick out, big, roomy, thin gums	○ Medium, soft, tender gums	○ Healthy, white, strong gums
SKIN	○ Thin, dry, cold, rough, dark	○ Smooth, oily, warm, rosy	○ Thick, oily, cool, white, pale
HAIR	○ Dry, brown, black, knotted brittle, scarce	○ Straight, oily, blond, gray, red, bald	○ Thick, curly, oily, wavy, luxuriant
NAILS	○ Dry, rough, brittle, break easily	○ Sharp, flexible, pink, lustrous	○ Thick, oily, smooth, polished
NECK	○ Thin, tall	○ Medium	○ Big, folded
CHEST	○ Flat, sunken	○ Moderate	○ Expanded, round
BELLY	○ Thin, flat, sunken	○ Moderate	○ Big, pot-bellied
BELLY BUTTON	○ Small, irregular, herniated	○ Oval, superficial	○ Big, deep, round, stretched
HIPS	○ Slender, thin	○ Moderate	○ Heavy, big
JOINTS	○ Cold, cracking	○ Moderate	○ Large, lubricated
APPETITE	○ Irregular, scanty	○ Strong, unbearable	○ Slow but steady
DIGESTION	○ Irregular, forms gas	○ Quick, causes burning	○ Prolonged, forms mucous
TASTE	○ Sweet, sour, salty	○ Sweet, bitter, astringent	○ Bitter, pungent, astringent
THIRST	○ Changeable	○ Surplus	○ Sparse
ELIMINATION	○ Constipation	○ Loose	○ Thick, oily, sluggish
Physical ACTIVITY	○ Hyperactive	○ Moderate	○ Slow
Mental ACTIVITY	○ Hyperactive	○ Moderate	○ Dull, slow
EMOTIONS	○ Anxiety, fear, uncertainty	○ Anger, hate, jealousy	○ Calm, greedy, attachment
FAITH	○ Variable	○ Extremist	○ Consistent
INTELLECT	○ Quick but faulty response	○ Accurate response	○ Slow, exact
RECOLLECTION	○ Recent good, remote poor	○ Distinct	○ Slow and sustained
DREAMS	○ Quick, active, many, fearful	○ Fiery, war, violence	○ Lakes, snow, romantic
SLEEP	○ Scanty, broken up, sleeplessness	○ Little but sound	○ Deep, prolonged
SPEECH	○ Rapid, unclear	○ Sharp, penetrating	○ Slow, monotonous
FINANCIAL	○ Poor, spends on trifles	○ Spends on luxuries	○ Rich, good money preserver
TOTALS	___ VATA	___ PITTA	___ KAPHA

THE AYURVEDIC INSTITUTE, 11311 MENAUL BLVD NE, ALBUQUERQUE, NM 87112-0008 · (505) 291-9698 · AYURVEDA.COM

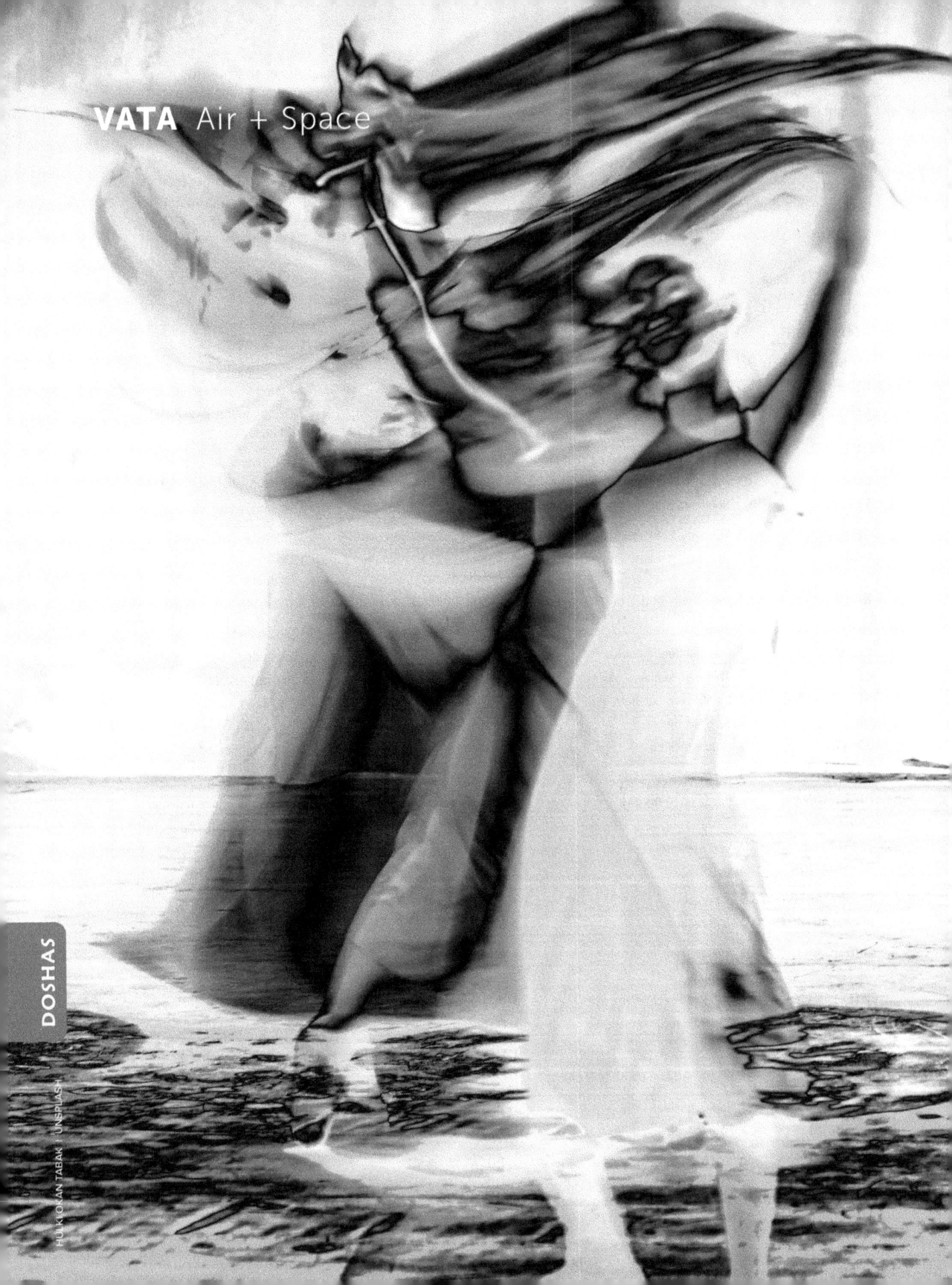

VATA Air + Space

DOSHAS

Vata Dosha is Movement

If we wanted to get the maximum health and wellness benefit from working with Ayurveda and we had to choose one Ayurvedic principle to understand and work with, that principle would be vata.

Of all three doshas vata has the most far-reaching effect in our body and in our life.

Vata dosha is a combination of air and space. Air is the dominant element in how vata functions in our body with space playing a supportive role. In exploring the air element in the section on the Five Elements (page 69), you were starting to get to know vata dosha.

VATA'S ELEMENTS
- Air
- Space

Life is movement and vata is the movement in our body. Nonstop movement is happening in every cell, tissue and organ in our body during every moment of our lives. This movement is the movement of our life-functions; it is the movement of vata dosha. Vata is a profoundly complex interplay of movement of different speeds, rhythms and qualities. Vata is the internal movement symphony that is keeping our body alive.

Our heart beats, our eyes blink and our nails grow. Food moves through our digestive tract, and blood flows through our veins and arteries. Thoughts move through our mind, emotions move through our body, and our body moves through space. Microscopic movement happens inside, around, and through the cells. And breathing, the grandmother of our movement, is an ever-present ebb and flow of breath moving in and out of our body; in and out of our cells. Our life and health rest on the intricate web of life-movement that is vata.

When we are balancing vata, we are helping to maintain harmony in this symphony. We are helping to keep the movement of the life-functions in our body running smoothly. In maintaining balanced vata we are supporting balance in the ever-shifting, delicate interplay of movement that is our life.

Understanding vata and its role in our body is essential for understanding Ayurveda and its application to yoga. Keeping vata balanced is the foundation of health.

Fortunately, keeping our vata in balance is less complicated than is vata itself. Daily asana practice and a little meditation go a long way in keeping ourselves healthy and maintaining balanced vata.

The gifts of vata are enthusiasm, creativity and joy. If we can truly keep our vata balanced, our health, happiness and well-being is assured.

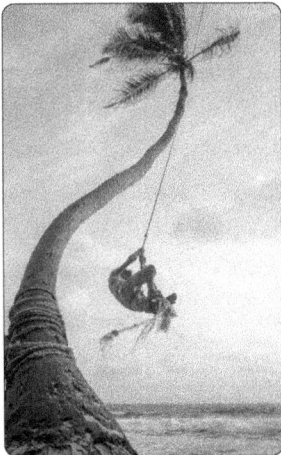

Qualities of Vata

Exploring a few of its qualities gives us more understanding of how vata functions in our body. Vata is cold, light and mobile. When vata is in balance, so too are these qualities. Some of the ways these qualities express themselves in our body/mind when they are balanced are:
- cool-headedness from the *cold* quality of vata
- light-heartedness from vata's *light* quality
- freedom of movement on all levels from vata's *mobile* quality.

When we have too much of one or more of these qualities, it means that our vata is disturbed. For example, the chill in our bones or the airy coolness in our body that often precedes getting the flu is an increase in the cold quality. Feeling light-headed, faint or ungrounded is an excess in vata's quality of lightness. When our mind is racing or we cannot settle physically or emotionally we have an excess of vata's mobile quality. A mild vata disturbance may express primarily through an increase in one quality, whereas in a strong vata disturbance, all three of these qualities will be increased.

Vata is movement, and as such it is always fluctuating. Mild vata imbalances are a normal and necessary part of our day. Necessary imbalances are expressions of the cyclical nature of the needs of our body and of our life. We cycle between being asleep and being awake, activity and rest, hunger and satiation, needing stimulation and needing quiet and

QUALITIES OF VATA
- Cold
- Light
- Mobile

DOSHAS

countless other normal imbalances that arise from this natural cycling. Our body communicates with us when we have been long enough in one part of a cycle and it is time to shift into the other part.

When we do not pay attention to and respond to these communications, a healthy imbalance starts down the road of becoming a problematic imbalance. How many times have we forgotten to eat lunch because we are too busy, and then found ourselves nauseated, tired, irritable and unable to enjoy the work of the afternoon?

We all miss these messages at times and, while it is not ideal, it is life. Making a habit of not paying attention to and responding to healthy imbalances, however, is setting the stage for stronger levels of vata disturbance. It is laying the foundation for poor health and disease.

In maintaining vata balance, we can take inspiration from wide-winged birds who sensitively ride the currants of air and glide effortless through the sky. They need only to make a subtle shift in the angle of their wings to receive ongoing support from the air. When we recognize a mild vata imbalance all it takes is a subtle shift to return us to balance and gracefully ride the currents of vata. This is the Ayurvedic art of maintaining balance.

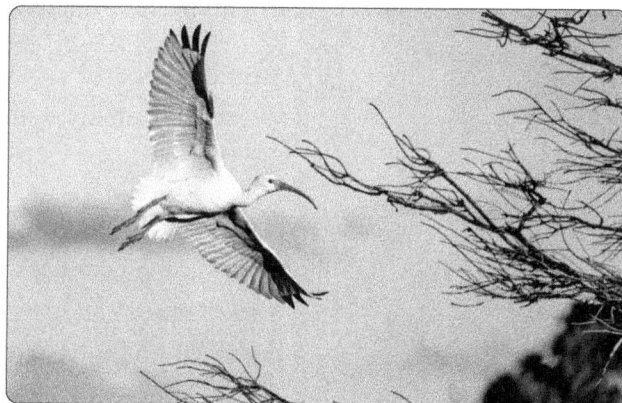

RICHARD SAGREDO | UNSPLASH

Keeping a gentle eye on our vata throughout the day allows us to catch the beginning of an imbalance. Having few antidotes at hand that we can easily apply lets us address that imbalance.

Vata balance is also the foundation for balance in the other two doshas. Awareness of our vata and a regular yoga practice goes a long way in keeping our life running smoothly.

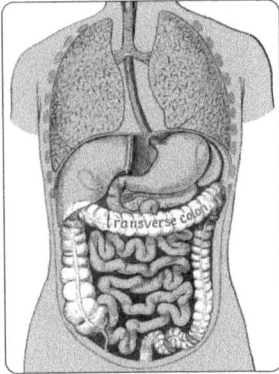

Vata's Home Site

The colon is the home site of vata and it is here where vata disturbance begins.

Regardless of which symptom(s) of disturbed vata we first notice, the disturbance itself begins in the colon with an increase in vata. For this reason, an asana practice that focuses on the colon, pelvis and lower abdomen is one of the go-to practices for vata balancing.

Abdominal gas, bloating or constipation are obvious expressions of an increase of vata. Other physical expressions of imbalanced vata are bumping into furniture, stumbling and tripping. Pushing our body to move faster than it is able to do so comfortably will create a vata disturbance. The reverse is also true, being vata-disturbed can propel us into pushing ourselves to do too much.

Mental/emotional signs of a vata disturbance are restlessness, hyperactivity and an inability to focus. Fear and anxiety are also speaking of a vata imbalance.

If we are able to notice and interrupt a mild vata disturbance, we can move through our days on an even keel and maintain stable health. It is easy to reverse an imbalance in its early stages — the trick is noticing it and having at hand ways to antidote the imbalance. When a disturbance becomes stronger and more complex, it can move beyond the colon and create problems throughout the body.

Strongly imbalanced vata actually pushes the other doshas into disturbance. We then have a pitta or kapha disturbance that was caused by disturbed vata. The symptoms of the pitta or kapha disturbance may then dominate our awareness, even though the root of the problem is in the disturbed vata. For this reason, we can never go wrong with a vata-balancing practice when we are out-of-sorts.

DOSHAS

A Simple Formula for a Vata-Soothing Practice

☞ Focus on aligning and stabilizing the pelvis.

☞ Choose 2 or 3 twists for alternating compression and release of the abdomen.

☞ Yield into and rest deeply in passive forward bends using head support. Any seated forward bend that you enjoy will do.

Clues for Recognizing Disturbed Vata

☞ Feeling spacey, fragmented or ungrounded.

☞ Having difficulty being still.

☞ Being constipated or having excess abdominal gas.

☞ Trying to do too many things.

☞ Experiencing unwarranted fear or anxiety.

☞ Feeling chilled, particularly if the temperature does not warrant it.

☞ Being mentally scattered or physically unstable.

On-the-Go Interventions for Balancing Vata

Having 3 or 4 favorite ways to antidote a vata disturbance makes it easier to know what to do when we recognize a disturbance developing. It's like having a vata-balancing first aid kit. We can also do preemptive vata balancing by doing 1 or 2 of these interventions every couple of hours.

☞ Pause, notice and enjoy something in your environment.

☞ Close your eyes, place your hand on your lower belly and feel the movement of your breathing.

☞ Do a forward bend from a standing position, letting the spine soften and release.

☞ Bring your attention to your breathing and gradually increase the length of your exhalations.

☞ Rest your forehead on your desk and feel the movement of your breathing in the lower abdomen.

☞ Sense your feet and wiggle your toes to increase sensation. You can do this seated or walking.

Getting in Touch with the Home Site of Vata - The Colon

☞ Clarify the shape and location of the colon by using your fingers to trace its outline on your torso.

☞ Lie on your stomach with a small folded towel under your abdomen. Sense the contact between the towel and your colon/lower abdomen.

☞ Rest in this position for a few minutes, feeling the movement of your breathing massaging this lower abdominal area.

☞ When your awareness is established in the lower abdomen, lift into a low cobra and stretch through the lower abdomen. Sense the increase in pressure between the abdomen and the towel.

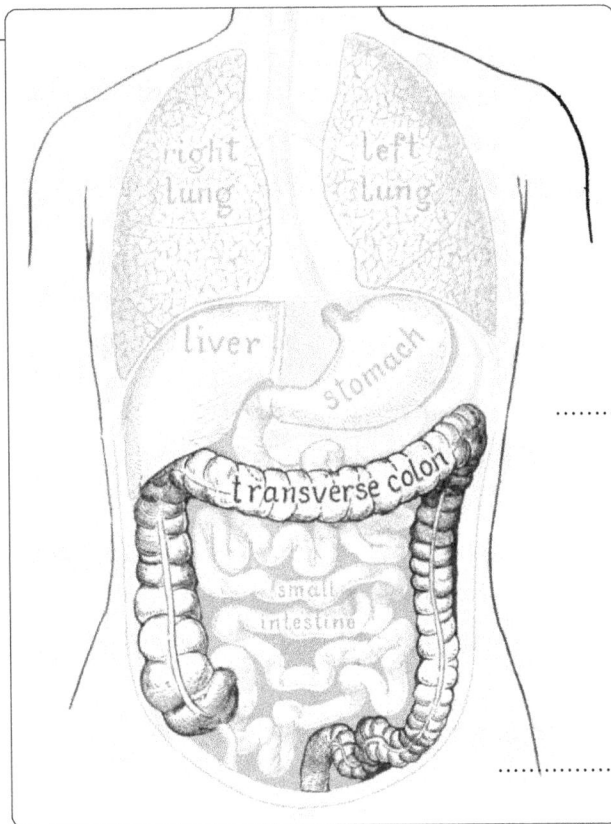

VATA HOME SITE
• COLON

DOSHAS

- Hold the pose as long as you comfortably can while focusing on the movement of your breath through the entire colon/lower abdomen.

- Very slowly release the cobra, sensing each part of the belly as it returns to its contact with the towel.

- Rest.

- Repeat 1 or 2 times.

- Lie on your back with your hands resting on the lower abdomen. Sense the movement of breath under your hands.

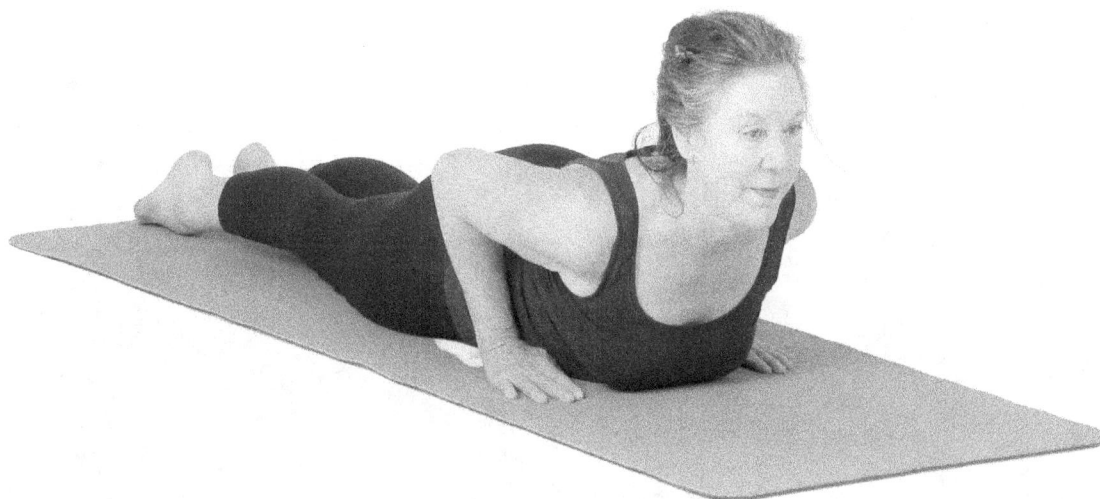

PITTA Fire + Water

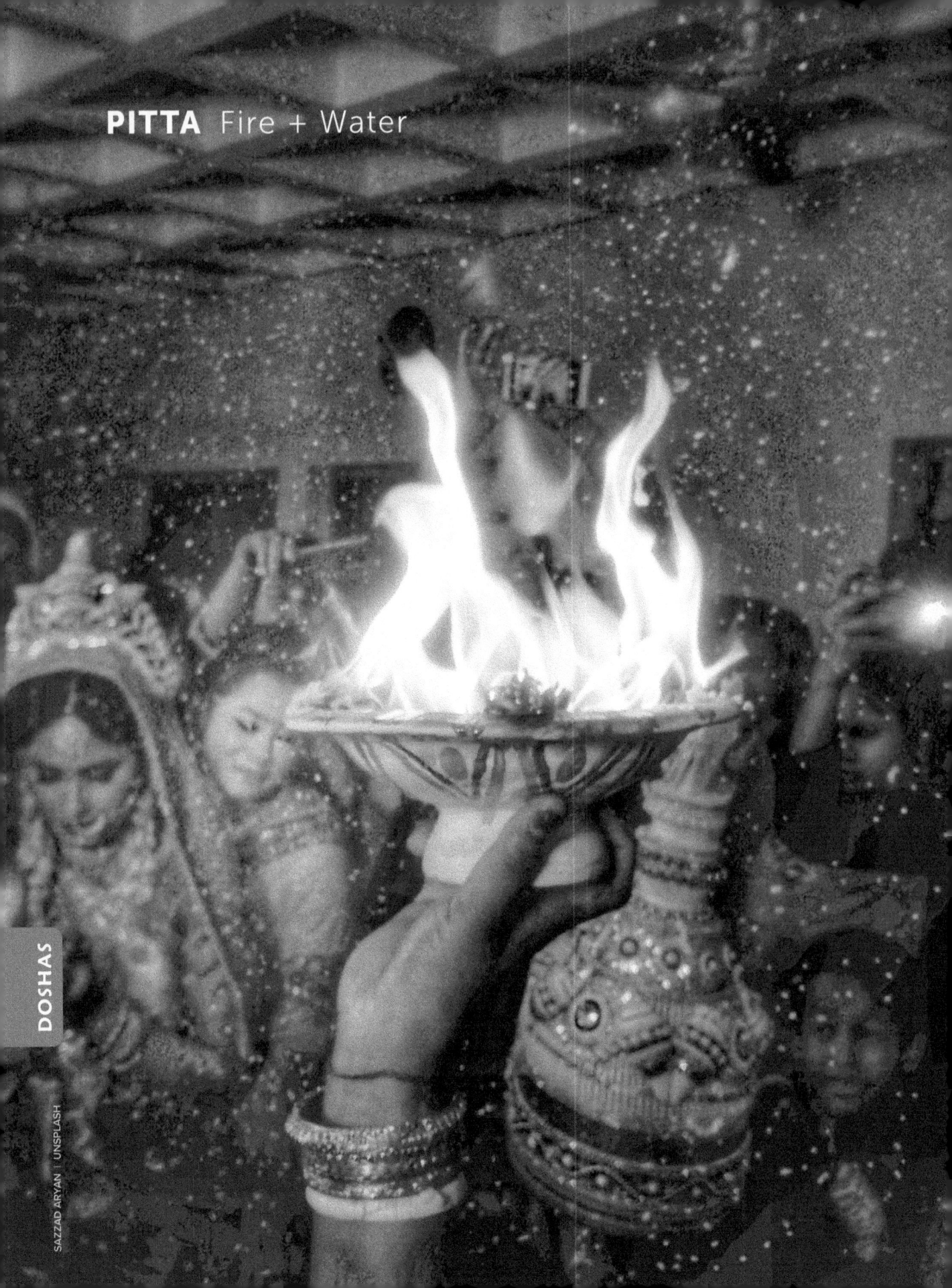

Pitta Dosha is Fire

Pitta is our biological fire. It heats, digests, consumes and transforms.

Pitta is the warmth in our heart and the brightness in our mind. Passion comes from pitta, whether is it is passion for a cause, for life, for creative endeavors, or a relationship. Glowing skin, sparkling eyes and radiance of mind, body or emotions, are expressing healthy pitta.

Pitta is our metabolism. It is through pitta's transformative power that we generate energy. Our stomach is a pot in which the food we eat is cooked by the fire of pitta so our body is able to absorb it. The nutrients from that food are further transformed into energy and into the tissues of our body. Delicious, healthy food serves us only to the degree that our internal fire can process it.

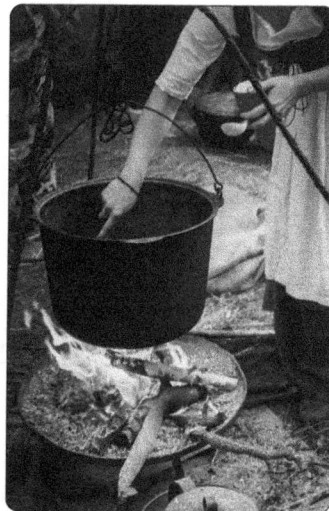

ARTEM MALTSEV | UNSPLASH

Pitta is a combination of fire and water with fire being the dominant element. Pitta's water is the carrier of pitta's fire. Pitta's water carries pitta's fire through the body and protects the body's tissues from being burnt by that fire. An example of this is the digestive enzymes and acids (pitta's fire) that are suspended in fluid (pitta's water). When this fluid mixes with the food that we eat, it also mixes the food with the digestive fire. Also, pitta's digestive fire would burn the tissues of the stomach were it not for the buffering action of the fluid in which it is carried.

PITTA'S ELEMENTS
- Fire
- Water

Our life is a creative journey involving the pitta-supported dynamics of learning, understanding and changing. Learning, understanding and changing are not separate things but rather are different facets of pitta's transformational power.

Changing negative thoughts, emotions and behaviors into positive ones is a process of transformation. It is through pitta's transforming energy that we convert anger into compassion, a disturbed mind into a peaceful one and resistance into acceptance.

Growing in wisdom involves the pitta-process of learning new ways of thinking and being; of freeing ourselves from the old and receiving the new. Pitta allows us to understand things in new ways. It is through pitta that words on a page become ideas in the mind, and that ideas in the mind become wisdom. It is through pitta that we digest our life experiences and use them to grow wiser. Pitta supplies the transforming energy that we need for living into our wholeness and discovering our potential.

Agni sara* is a yoga practice that enlivens digestive fire. It is a good practice for stimulating pitta but it has some important contraindications and so is best learned from a teacher.

As we age, our pitta weakens and so too does our capacity for digestion, assimilation and transformation. This dimming of our pitta results in a reduced ability to process food, to assimilate new ideas and to enjoy new experiences.

Keeping pitta strong and healthy is key to remaining vital, healthy and engaged with life as we age.

Qualities of Pitta

We can get to know pitta better by looking at its qualities and how they express in our body/mind. Pitta is hot, sharp and light. The hot quality of pitta gives heat to our body. It gives us emotional warmth and it is the underlying energy of passion in the body, mind and heart.

QUALITIES OF PITTA
- Hot
- Sharp
- Light

Pitta's sharp quality gives us a *sharp* mind. Our ability to see and to know something clearly happens through the *illuminating* power of pitta's light. Balanced pitta gives us perceptual clarity, precision of focus and the discriminating capacity to make skillful choices.

When pitta is balanced, its qualities are also balanced. When pitta is disturbed, pitta's qualities increase. A pitta disturbance expressing as an increase in the hot quality creates heated emotions like anger, frustration and impatience. An increase in the *sharp* quality of pitta makes us sharp-tongued, irritable and edgy. Pitta's *light* quality, when it is in excess, can create an intensified clarity of perception that is hard-edged and

see Appendix, page 230

inflexible. This hard-edged and inflexible quality makes it difficult to use this clarity in a cooperative and caring way.

By recognizing that these emotions and responses are excess pitta, we can relate to them differently than we otherwise would. Instead of wrestling with the emotions and responses themselves, we can focus our attention on antidoting the excess heat in our body/mind that is fueling them.

Focusing on reducing pitta rather than trying to control the disturbed emotions themselves gives us a tiny bit of emotional space. That tiny space is sufficient to allow us to choose how to respond to our inner experience rather than reacting from it. We have the *space* to choose to move toward compassion and equanimity rather than irritability and anger.

Disturbed pitta expresses itself physically in rashes, burning in the stomach, prickly skin, feeling overheated, unquenchable appetite, nausea and diarrhea. Any inflammation is excess pitta.

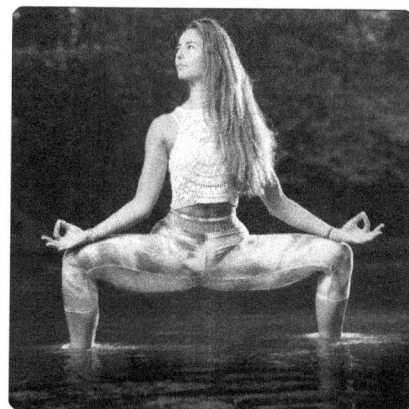

RAPHAEL NAST | UNSPLASH

A focus on grounding and connecting to earth is a good starting place for using asana to balance pitta. Pittas tend to be active, externally oriented people who are attracted to vigorous asana practice. Meditative asana, while less natural to pitta people, is very useful for pitta balancing because of its cooling and soothing benefits. It is important for pittas to keep in mind that always pushing to their maximum physical, mental or emotional capacity is pitta disturbing.

ELEMENTS FOR REDUCING PITTA

• Earth
• Water

Being in or otherwise engaging nature is important for keeping pitta balanced. Doing yoga outside in a shaded area, having plants in a practice space and using nature imagery in asana are ways of engaging nature's energy in yoga practice.

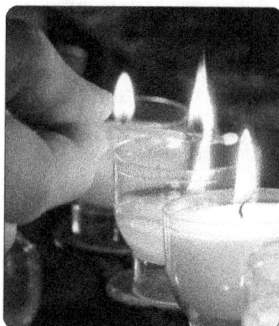

PIXEL2013 | PIXABAY

Agni is the Hindu god of fire. Externally he expresses as the sun, internally he is our body's heat. Agni burns away all impurities allowing us to access our innate radiance. Temples in India that are dedicated to Agni keep a flame burning day and night. Contemplating this image may inspire us to remember the importance of tending our inner fire.

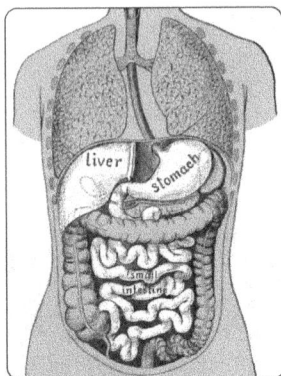

Pitta's Home Site

The home site of pitta is in the stomach, liver and small intestine.

If you enjoy anatomical detail, clarifying the position, size and shape of the individual pitta organs can be a way of developing self-awareness. You can also use that anatomical clarity to direct the action of asana or the movement of breath.

If you are not so inclined to learn about anatomical detail, it is not a problem. It can be equally effective to focus on the upper abdomen between the bottom of the breastbone and the navel, and the center of the lower abdomen. Putting your awareness inside the body rather than just on the surface more fully engages the pitta organs.

Regardless of how you notice a pitta disturbance, it is important to remember that the disturbance itself starts in pitta's home site. Pitta's home site is a primary area of focus in balancing pitta, whether for creating a practice devoted to pitta-balancing, or for bringing a little pitta-balancing into a regular practice. An easy and effective way to encourage pitta balance in its home site is softening the abdomen.

Lightly resting one palm on the upper abdomen over the stomach and liver area, and the other palm on the center of the lower abdomen over the small intestine attracts the breath to these areas. Sensing the movement of your breathing under the palms and through the pitta organs while encouraging a velvet-like softness in the breath relaxes both the abdominal muscles and pitta organs. In doing so, disturbed pitta is soothed. Another version of this is focusing on the weight of the hands or the warmth of the palms on the abdomen while sensing the hands being moved by the breath.

Spending a few minutes softening the abdominal muscles and pitta organs in this manner is a good way to start a pitta-balancing practice. You can then check in with your abdomen periodically throughout the practice to help it remember that softness.

This is a pleasant and easy antidote for disturbed pitta that can be integrated into any yoga practice, or into a few moments that you carve out for yourself in a busy day.

A Simple Formula for a Pitta-Soothing Practice

Lie on your back with your palm resting on your upper abdomen and connect to your breath and pitta organs as described on previous page.

Do a couple of simple **Reclining Twists**, *gently* focusing their spiraling action into pitta's home site. Use two different twists, or one twist repeated twice. You can use **Seated Twists** if you prefer.

End with a supported **Seated Forward Bend** using a head support and long, relaxed exhalations. Any Forward Bend that you enjoy is effective.

Clues for Recognizing Disturbed Pitta

- Reactivity and quickness to anger.
- Feeling overly driven.
- Being critical or judgmental.
- Irritability and impatience.
- Hyper-acidity, heartburn or fever.
- Strong desire to eat without being hungry.
- Excess heat; mentally, physically or emotionally.

On-the-Go Interventions for Balancing Pitta

- Use the power of imagination. Imagine being by a waterfall and feeling its cooling spray; alternately, choose one of your favorite cooling nature spots.
- Exhale through the feet and into the earth.
- With palm resting on the upper abdomen just below the breastbone, connect to the movement of the breath.
- Elongate the exhalation and shorten the inhalation.
- Do cooling pranayamas — Sitali and Sitkari.*
- Lean upper back against a wall (or a tree) and yield into that support. Breathe in and out through the back of the heart.
- Use any of the vata on-the-go antidotes on page 101. Remember that disturbed vata often pushes pitta into disturbance.

*see Appendix, page 229

Getting in Touch with the Home Site of Pitta - The Stomach, Liver and Small Intestine

- Clarify the shape and location of the stomach, liver and small intestine by tracing their outline on your torso with your fingers. Be aware of their three-dimensionality.

- Sit with your right palm resting on the area of your liver and, with a meditative mind, sense your breath moving into and softening all three dimensions of the liver. Stay with this for a minute or so.

- Sit with your left palm resting on the area of your stomach and, with a meditative mind, sense your breath moving into and softening all three dimensions of the stomach. Stay with this for a minute or so.

- Repeat this process with a palm resting on the center of your lower abdomen over the small intestine.

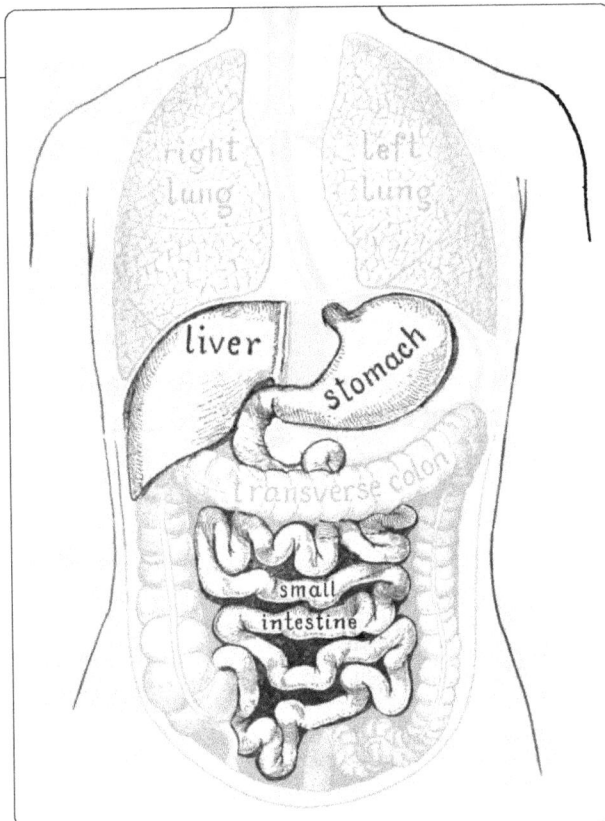

PITTA HOME SITE
- STOMACH
- LIVER
- SMALL INTESTINE

DOSHAS

- ∿ Come into **Seated Spinal Twist** to the right. As you hold the twist sense your breath moving through the liver. Hold for a minute or so.

- ∿ Release the pose slowly, being aware of the un-spiraling movement through the liver.

- ∿ Come into **Seated Spinal Twist** to the left. As you hold the twist sense your breath moving through the stomach. Hold for a minute or so.

- ∿ Release the pose slowly, being aware of the un-spiraling movement through the stomach.

- ∿ Rest in sitting or in **Savasana**, being aware of the movement of your breathing through the upper abdomen and pitta organs.

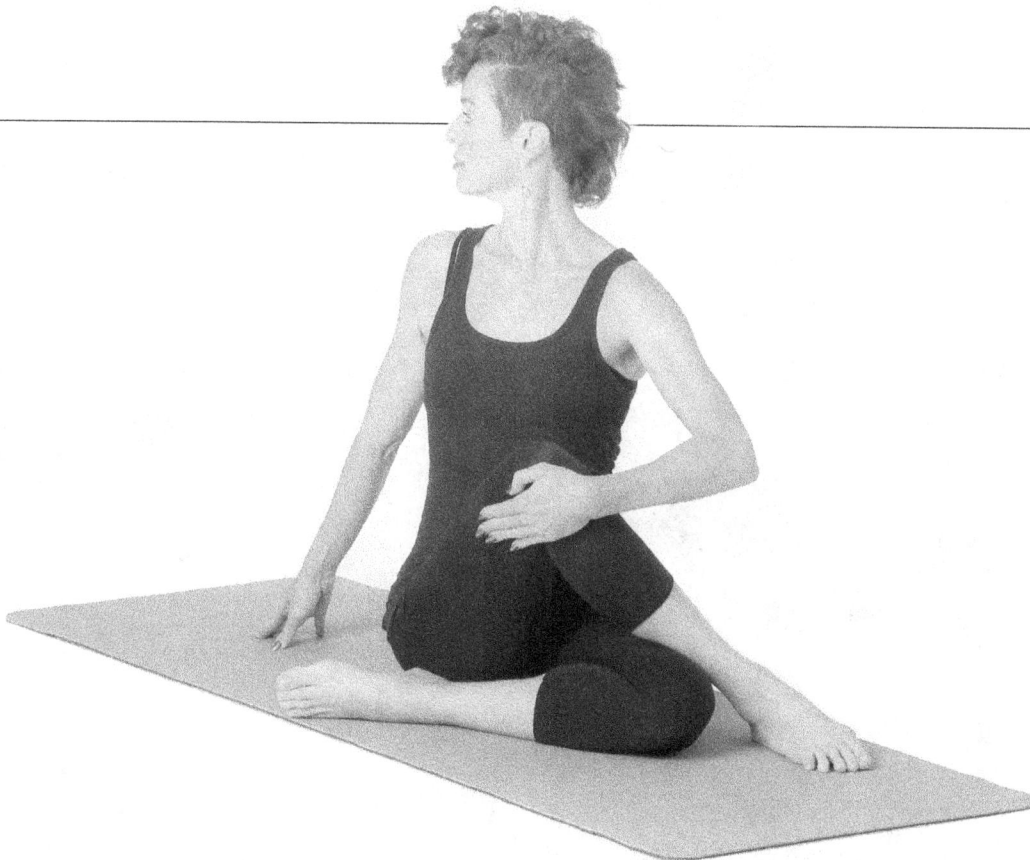

KAPHA Earth + Water

Kapha Dosha is Substance

Kapha is a combination of earth and water. Kapha gives us substance, shape and form. Everything about ourselves that we can see and touch is kapha.

Balanced kapha is like a steadfast friend supporting us in everything we do, including helping us to keep pitta and vata in balance.

Earth is the dominant element in kapha and is the primary substance of the structure of the body. The water element supports the structure of the body and plays a key role in its function. Unlike the discussion of pitta and vata, the discussion of kapha looks at both the earth and water aspects. While pitta and vata are also a combination of two elements, their dominant element is significantly more dominant and so is more relevant for its application to yoga practice.

KAPHA'S ELEMENTS
• Earth
• Water

People with a kapha constitution are considered fortunate because they tend to have strong bodies and stable health. Kaphas have greater endurance than do pittas and vatas and they can more easily maintain balanced vata. Since vata imbalance is the root cause of most health problems, this puts kapha ahead of the game for staying healthy.

Kapha expresses itself on a continuum from solid to fluid. Bones are on the earthy/solid end of that continuum. Muscles and organs express themselves on a range of greater or lesser solidity/fluidity depending on the muscle or organ itself and its state of health. On the watery end of kapha's solid/fluid continuum are tears, saliva, blood and protective fluids.

The watery aspect of kapha cleanses, nourishes and protects. Joints move easily and without pain because they are protected by synovial fluid. Lungs move freely in the ribcage during breathing because they are lubricated with pleural fluid. Blood carries nourishment to, and cleanses waste products from the cells. The brain and spinal cord are suspended in and protected by cerebrospinal fluid.

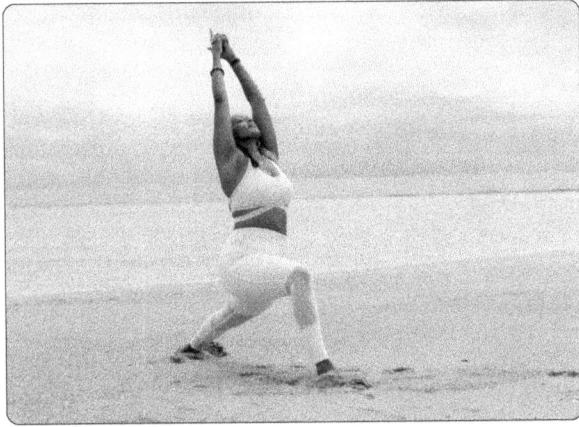

Asana directly engages the kapha aspect of the body through the wide variety of actions created by different asanas. Asana stimulates, massages, stretches, shapes, enlivens and mobilizes our substance/body, both its earthy and its fluid aspects. This keeps our body healthy, vital and responsive. It keeps our kapha solid but not too solid, and fluid but not too fluid.

Vinyasa, both vigorous and meditative, is valuable for kapha balancing. A vigorous vinyasa is heating and so it stimulates kapha with both heat and movement. A meditative vinyasa softens kapha's hardness, lightens kapha's density and mobilizes kapha's tendency to be static. A meditative vinyasa needs to be done for at least thirty minutes in order to have a kapha-balancing effect.

All vinyasas are useful for cultivating healthy movement and encouraging a balanced flow in the fluids of the body. Since balanced flow is one of the definitions of health, awakening the fluids of the body with vinyasa practice is an important contribution to kapha balancing.

Squeeze-and-engorge is an aspect of asana practice that is particularly beneficial for kaphas. Squeeze-and-engorge is a process in which one part of the body is pressed firmly into another part of the body. The point of this is to create a strong compressive action that squeezes the fluid out of the area being compressed. When the pose is released, that area of the body is then flooded with fresh blood. This happens naturally in some asanas. We can also actively cultivate this process in asana, and use it as a focus around which to organize a kapha-balancing practice.

The pressure used in squeeze-and-engorge mechanically breaks down the excess density of kapha. Deep twisting actions that use this process to focus on the thoracic spine are a good way to stimulate the home site of kapha.

As a general rule, vitalizing and stimulating the body are key for maintaining balanced kapha.

DOSHAS

The Qualities of Kapha

We can get to know kapha in more detail through its qualities. Dense, stable, heavy and static are qualities that kapha gets from its earth aspect. Soft, smooth and cohesive are qualities that kapha gets from its water aspect.

Kapha people make good friends because they are patient and easy-going. Their earthy qualities make them reliable, steady and predictable so they are there when you need them. Kapha's water qualities give them a loving, gentle and compassionate nature.

When kapha's earth qualities are out of balance we become excessively dense, heavy, and static. This excess in kapha's earth aspect restricts the flow of life energies in the body which sets the stage for stagnation.

On the psychological level, an increase in kapha's heaviness and density creates heaviness in the mind and emotions. We become stubborn, dull and lethargic. Depression is a common result. This type of kapha imbalance makes it hard for us to get ourselves moving, and makes it difficult for us to stay engaged with life.

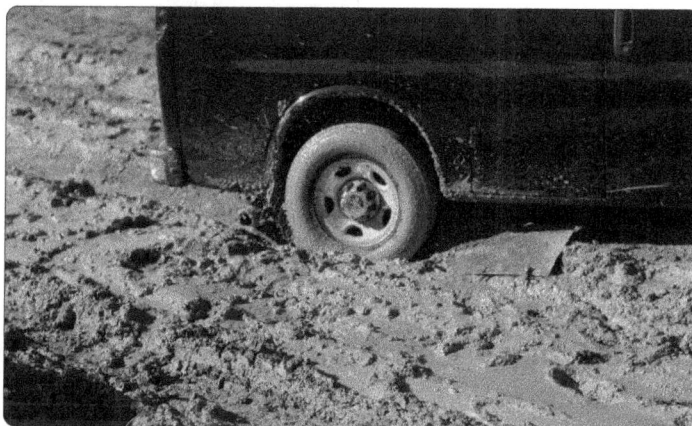

AUBREY ROSE ODOM | UNSPLASH

Imbalanced kapha expressing through its water qualities makes us too watery or too sticky. We are familiar with this from having a cold. Sometimes during a cold our mucus becomes so thin that it drips from our nose. At other times during a cold an excess in the cohesive quality of kapha expresses itself as a sticky congestion in the lungs or sinuses. Disturbed kapha in its water aspect also expresses as water retention and swelling.

Psychologically, excess water makes it hard for us to hold to a point of view or to stand up for ourselves. We have difficulty settling on a clear direction in life, setting boundaries and making decisions. Clinginess and possessiveness can be flavors of a kapha imbalanced in its water aspect.

Physically, an excess in the water aspect of kapha leaves our body too watery. One of the results can be a loss of musculoskeletal integrity which can result in physical sloppiness.

When they are imbalanced, kapha people tend to gain weight and become heavier and denser, or heavier and waterier. Both of these expressions of kapha imbalance suppress the vitality of pitta and vata and so block our access to vata's lightness and pitta's brightness.

Disturbed kapha creates stagnation and congestion in the body. Stagnation and congestion set the stage for poor health because the tissues and organs become bogged down and cannot function optimally.

Kapha needs regular activity and strong stimulation to express the best of its nature. All vinyasas, particularly vigorous ones, benefit kapha because they mobilize earth and support balanced flow. Inversions, Hero poses and balance poses are all good choices to keep kapha balanced, as is the challenge of learning new poses.

Kapha's Home Site

The home site of kapha dosha is in the lungs. It is here where a kapha disturbance begins. This is true regardless of where and how we first recognize the disturbance. As the home site of kapha, attention to opening and stimulating the lungs, neck and the area just below the diaphragm should be included in any kapha-balancing practice.

Heaviness or congestion in any part of kapha's home site indicates an increase in kapha. If our stomach feels full a half hour or more after eating, we can suspect a kapha imbalance. Lethargy, sleeping too much, emotional heaviness, lack of interest in life, depression and feeling like it is too much effort to move our body are all signs of kapha disturbance.

Any practice that heats the body and raises the heart rate helps to liquefy, mobilize and cleanse the body of excess kapha. Backbends are good for stretching through and stimulating kapha's home site, while Twists can be used to create a wringing action through the thoracic spine and lungs. The movement and intensified breathing in a vigorous vinyasa practice is particularly helpful for kapha balancing.

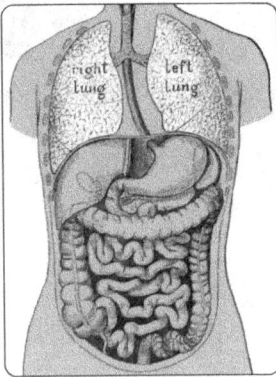

ELEMENTS FOR BALANCING WATER & EARTH

- Fire
- Air

A Simple Formula for a Kapha-Balancing Practice

◎ Choose 2 or 3 **Backbends** and a couple of **Hero** poses.

◎ Focus on stretching through the arms, enlivening the upper spine and opening the ribcage.

◎ Emphasize an elongated inhalation, either equal to or longer than the exhalation.

Clues for Recognizing Disturbed Kapha

◎ Congested lungs, throat or sinuses.

◎ Heaviness in the stomach.

◎ Feeling full an hour or more after eating.

◎ Holding tenaciously to the past.

◎ Feeling sluggish and lethargic.

◎ Depression.

◎ Excess resistance and stubbornness.

◎ Accepting things out of passivity.

On-the-Go Interventions for Balancing Kapha

◎ Stretch arms overhead to stimulate and open the ribcage.

◎ 4 or 5 elongated inhalations to lift and expand the chest, spread the breastbone and widen the shoulder girdle.

◎ 4 or 5 elongated inhalations to open the ribcage front to back, side to side and top to bottom.

◎ Extend one arm above your head then side bend to open the ribcage. Repeat on the other side.

◎ Bastrika* breathing: Rapid inhalations and exhalations of equal lengths. 20 breaths, rest for 5 then repeat.

◎ Elongated inhalations together with shortened exhalations.

see Appendix, page 228

Getting in Touch with the Home Site of Kapha - The Lungs

◎ Lie on your back, taking a minute or so for your body to settle and your mind to turn inward.

◎ Explore the shape and location of your lungs by using your fingers to trace their outline on your body. Note that the top of the lungs come a little bit above the collar bones.

◎ With fingers spread, lay your hands on your chest as if to lay them on as much of your lungs as possible. Breathe into the fronts of the lungs by breathing toward the sensation of your hands on your chest. Continue long enough to awaken the sensation of the fronts of your lungs.

◎ Put your right hand on the side of your upper left ribcage just below the armpit to awaken the side of the left lung. Breathe into the side of the left lung by directing your breath toward the sensation of your hand. Repeat this process by putting your left hand on the right side of your ribcage.

◎ With your arms alongside your body, breathe into the sides of your lungs. Continue long enough to awaken the sensation of simultaneously breathing into sides of both lungs.

KAPHA HOME SITE
• LUNGS

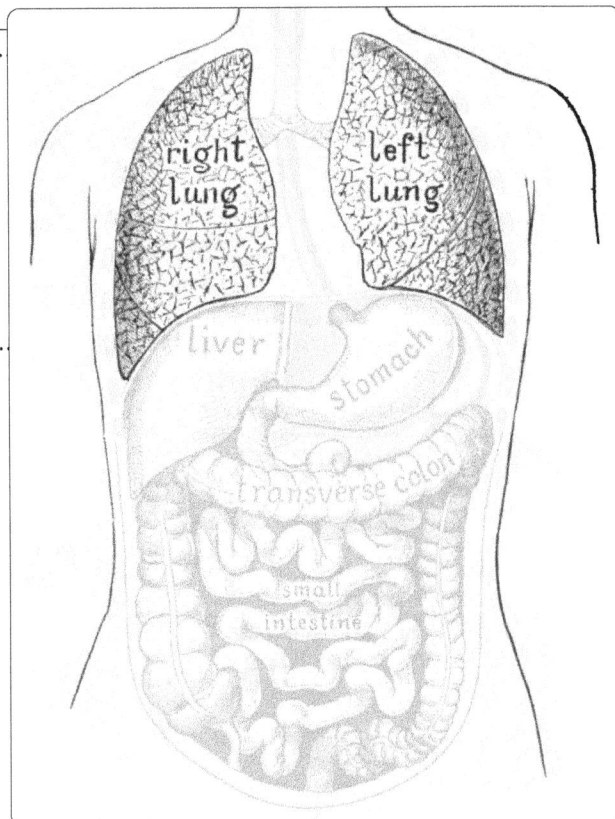

- ◎ Be aware of the back of the lungs by sensing the contact of your upper back on the floor. Breathe into the backs of the lungs.

- ◎ Rest for a few moments and sense yourself breathing in the entire three-dimensionality of the lungs.

- ◎ Maintain awareness of the lungs as you come into **Fish** pose. Notice which area of the lungs are automatically enlivened by the pose. Expand the length, width and depth of your ribcage and use your inhalations to awaken aliveness in different areas of the lungs.

- ◎ Rest briefly in **Savasana**, then repeat the pose.

- ◎ Return to **Savasana** and become aware of the movement of your lungs as you breathe. Without interfering or judging, notice the areas of your lungs in which the breath flows easily and the areas in which it does not.

- ◎ Rest as long as you like.

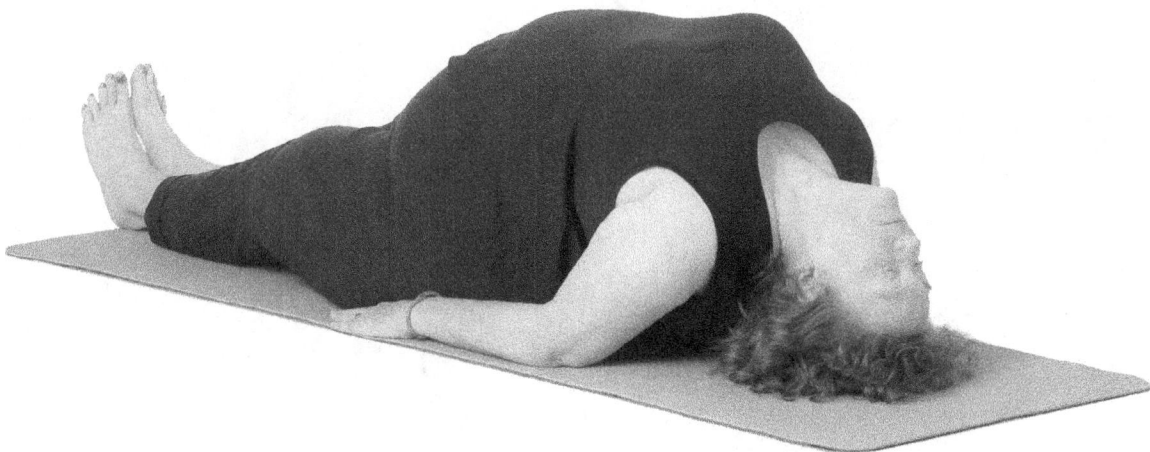

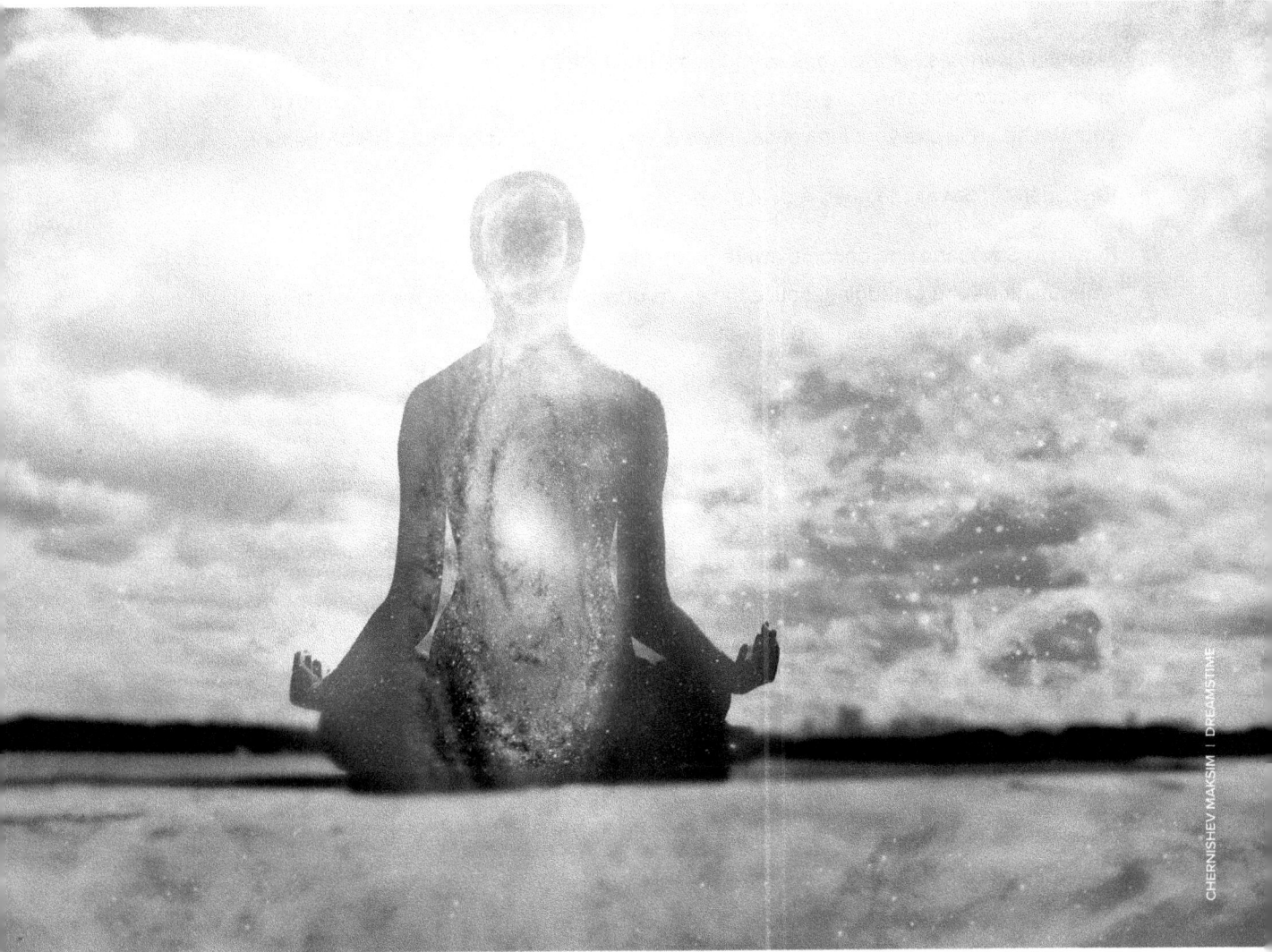

CHERNISHEV MAKSIM | DREAMSTIME

What Is Prana?

Prana is our life energy. It underlies everything that we are and everything that we do. It permeates our entire body and the space around it.

Prana is a subtle aspect of the air element. Yoga and Ayurveda both see prana as essential to achieving their respective goals.

Yoga works with prana indirectly through asana practice, and directly through pranayama. The various pranayamas are designed for regulating, refining, stabilizing and awakening prana. Ayurveda engages prana through its healing protocols, which include yoga practices.

The following chapters discuss the **five major directions** in which prana flows through our body, along with descriptions of the physiological functions and musculoskeletal actions that each direction of pranic flow supports. Understanding the structures and functions supported by each of the five pranas is the basis of using them in yoga practice for balancing the doshas.

Breath and prana are closely related so breathing is our easiest access into working with prana in yoga practice.

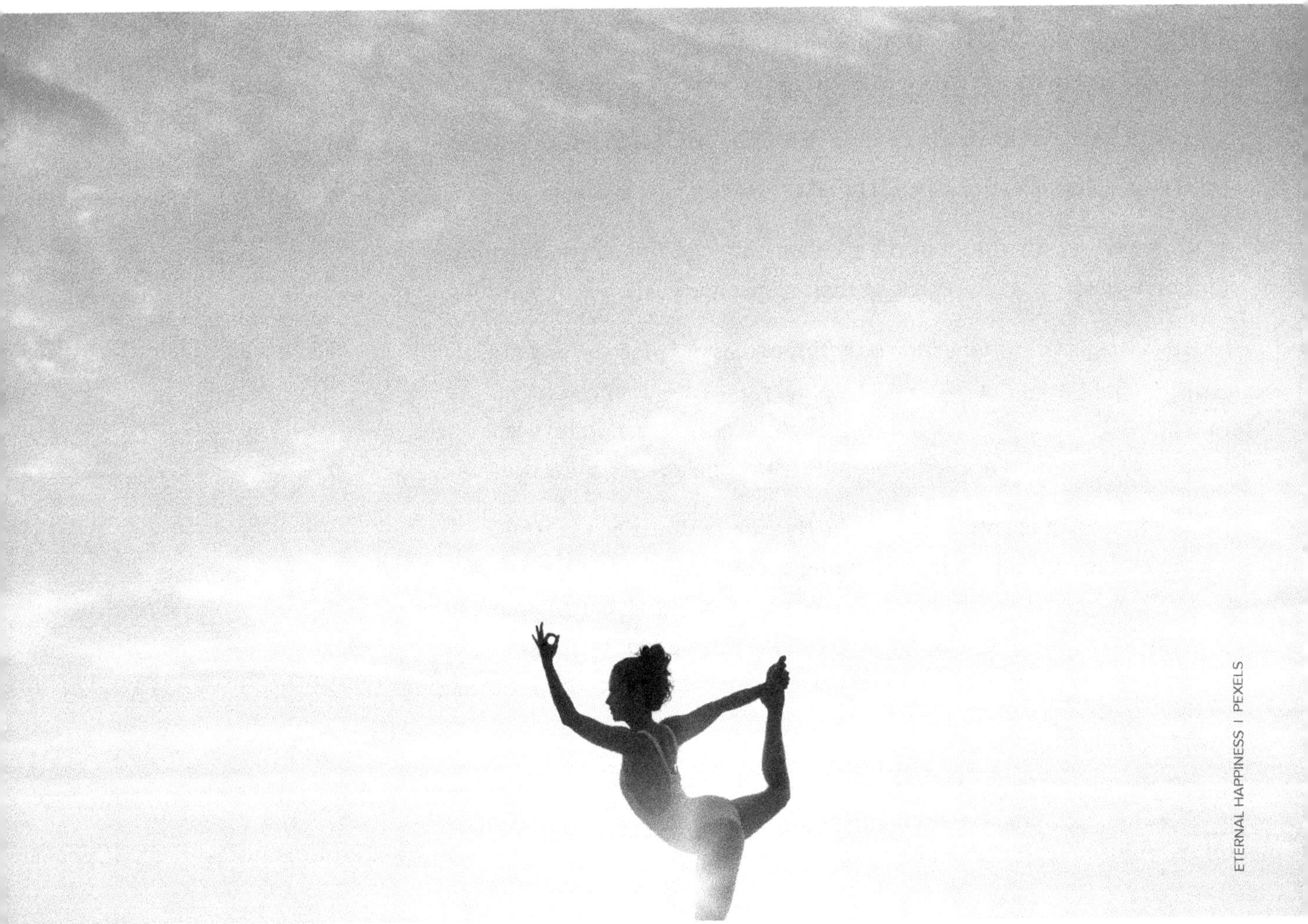

ETERNAL HAPPINESS | PEXELS

PRANA

Entering the World of Prana

In talking about prana and the body, Swami Veda Bharati would use an analogy of a magnet and iron filings. When a U-shaped magnet is placed below a table on which there are iron filings, the iron filings gather around the energy field of the magnet, taking on its U-shaped form.

Just as iron filings take on the shape of a magnetic field, so, too, our muscles, organs and tissues organize around pranic fields. When our prana is balanced, healthy and clear, so too is our body.

Asana and Prana

Prana and the body are a two-way street. In working with prana we are working with the underlying energy of physical actions. The reverse is also true. In working with physical actions of asana, we are creating pathways of pranic flow.

We can work separately with prana and the body, but in working with one we are necessarily working with the other. Clarifying asanas and prana separately lets us work more effectively with them together.

Asanas in which we have ease and confidence have good pranic support. Asanas in which we are lacking ease and confidence are lacking good pranic support. When we are challenged by an asana, it is helpful to alternate our focus between its musculoskeletal actions and its underlying prana.

All of this being said, we can work with our body in a way that actually disrupts the relationship between our physical and pranic bodies. During asana practice, cultivating whole-body awareness and allowing natural breathing goes a long way to supporting a harmonious relationship between the physical and pranic bodies.

When we are challenged by an asana, it is helpful to alternate our focus between its musculoskeletal actions and its underlying prana.

What are the Five Pranas?

Prana flows through our body in five directions. When talking about the Five Pranas we are talking about directions of pranic flow, not five different pranas. There is only one prana.

Prana and its five major directions of flow are important in both Ayurveda and yoga. While yoga refers to the *five pranas*, Ayurveda talks about the *five vayus* or the *five subdoshas of vata.* All of these terms are referring to the same thing. For simplicity sake we will use the yogic term, the Five Pranas.

Another point of confusion is that one of the five pranas is called *prana.* So, the term prana is used both for prana itself, *and* also for one of the directions of pranic flow in our body. We can think about these as being big prana and little pranas — like the ocean and the waves. The five directions of pranic flow are little pranas or waves, and big prana is prana itself.

––––––––––––––––––––

Each of the five pranas influences the whole body but has its primary effect in the area of the body in which it moves. In getting to know the pranas individually we are also getting to know the body structures and functions that each pranic flow supports.

The five pranas function together as a dynamic interplay with each being dependent on the other. If one prana is particularly weak or particularly strong it is so, in part, because of its relationship with the other pranas. Although all of the pranas are interrelated, some pranas are more closely related.

When cultivating one of the five pranas, we want to keep in mind that the different pranic flows are waves of a single prana. Sometimes we can have difficulty awakening one direction of pranic flow only to have it spontaneously appear as we are working with a different prana. If we are having difficulty accessing one of the pranas, it is helpful to explore it in relation to the others.

PRANA

The five pranas can be used for cultivating whole-body integration, supporting coordination and augmenting muscular strength. The pranas also have much to contribute to specific wellness goals like improving sleep, strengthening digestion and even things like supporting the healing of a broken bone. Clear, vital pranic flow supports the health of all of the body structures and functions through which it flows.

Prana has often been described as a *subtle energy inside the breath*. Breath awareness is the doorway into connecting with prana. Working with the breath is how we refine prana and engage it for Ayurvedic balancing.

"To bring about positive transformations in body and mind we must understand the energy through which they work. This force is called prana in Sanskrit, meaning 'primary energy,' sometimes translated as 'breath' or 'vital force'."

— David Frawley

PRANA
down and in

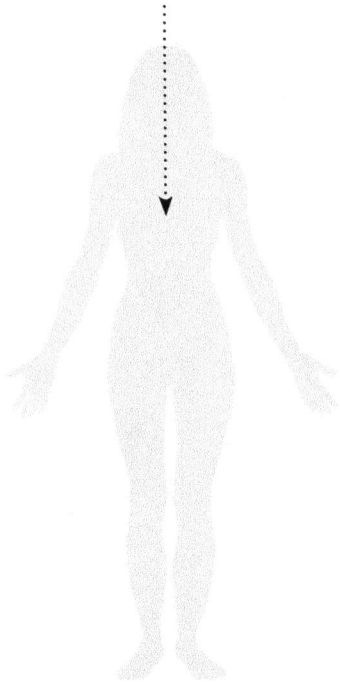

UDANA
up and out

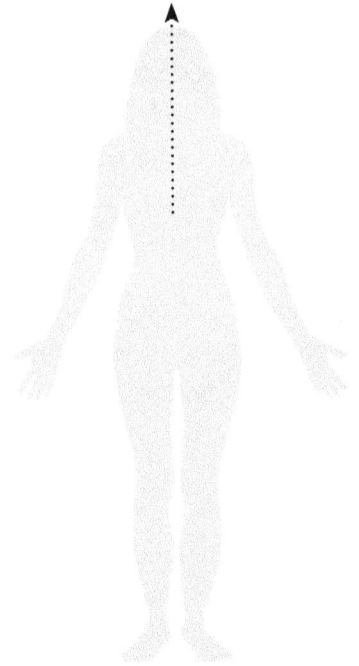

APANA
down and out

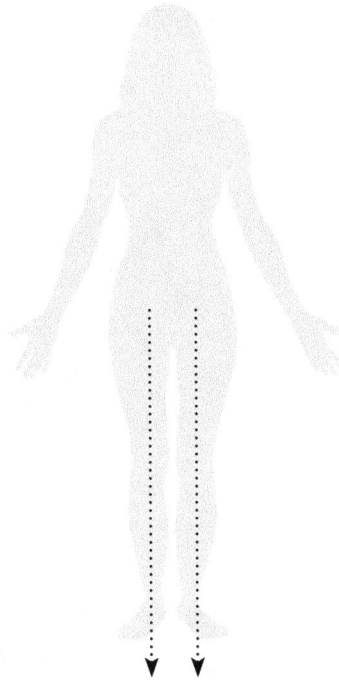

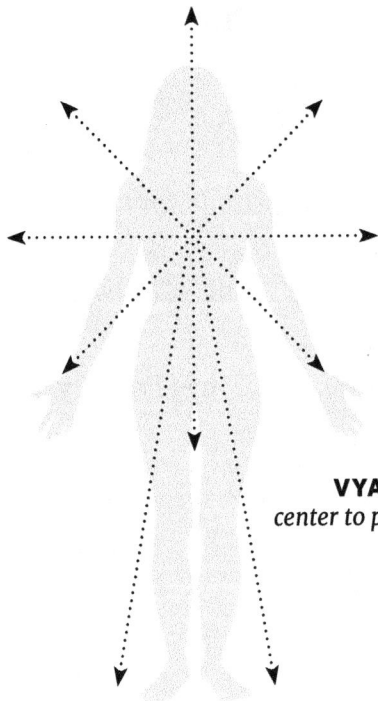

VYANA
center to periphery

SAMANA
periphery to center

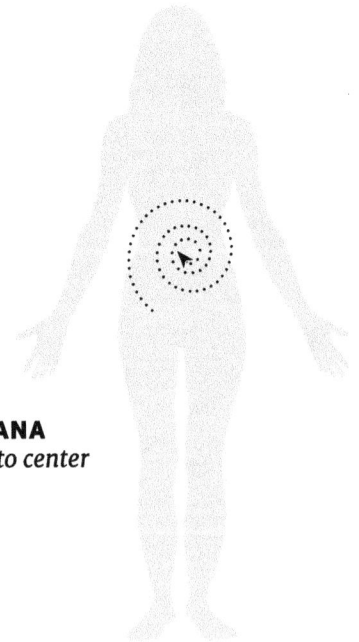

PRANA

Getting to Know the Five Pranas

In working with the Five Pranas, the following practices use breathing, imagery and sensation.

People vary as to whether sensation or imagery comes more easily to them. Either sensing or imaging or a combination of both are fine for working with the pranas. The important thing is being clear about the directions of pranic flow and connecting awareness of that flow to the movement of the breath.

The five directions of pranic flow are:

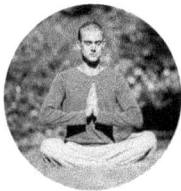

PRANA:
down and in

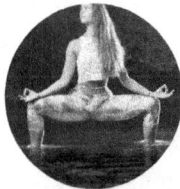

APANA:
down and out

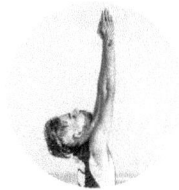

UDANA:
up and out

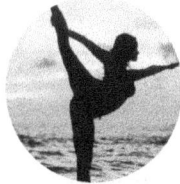

VYANA:
center to periphery

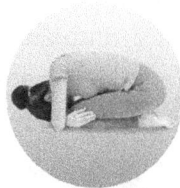

SAMANA:
periphery to center

Prana

PRANA

- Down and In
- Crown to Diaphragm
- Balanced by Udana

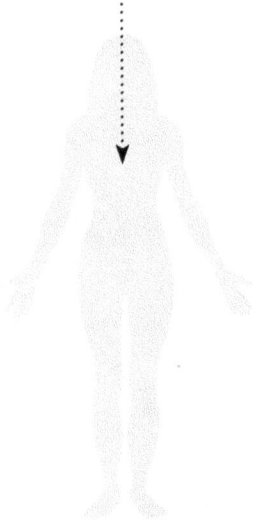

Prana flows inward and downward. It enters into the body through the crown of the head and flows downward through the head, neck and chest, into the area of the heart. Prana is the energetic support for inhaling. Everything that we take into ourselves from the outside world we do so with the support of prana.

Prana serves as an energetic umbilical cord through which we connect to and receive nourishment from the universe.

Clarity of mind is more available to us when we have a healthy flow of prana through the head. Clear pranic flow through the head, neck and chest enhances communication between the heart and the mind — a heart-informed mind and a mind-informed heart enhances every area of our life.

A well-coordinated upper body requires integrated movement of the head, neck and torso. This integration happens with the support of prana. It is through clear prana that we are able to enjoy freedom through the arms and shoulders, ease through the neck, and vitality in the chest. Prana is important for safely doing inversions.

Tension anywhere in the head, neck and chest can restrict the flow of prana. Common spots of tension through this area are around the eyes and inside the eye sockets, the jaw, the tongue, the throat and the transition area between the neck and chest. Softening and letting go of tension in these areas helps to free pranic flow. The reverse is also true. Cultivating prana encourages a release of tension in these areas.

Everything that we take into ourselves from the outside world we do so with the support of prana.

Inhaling, swallowing, sucking and eating are all functions of prana. The flow of air into the nose, down through the windpipe and into the lungs rides on the flow of prana — as does food entering the mouth and moving down through the esophagus and into the stomach. People with respiratory problems or eating disorders may benefit by an intensive practice of awakening prana.

Taking in ideas and experiences are also functions of prana. When we can't *swallow something*, our prana is not flowing freely. Anytime we have difficulty taking something in, whether it is food, breath, ideas, feelings or life experience, giving attention to prana is helpful.

Symptoms of imbalanced prana include insomnia, low energy and mental hyperactivity. Unstable, unreliable energy can also be caused by imbalanced prana.

Cultivating pranic flow is done most easily in combination with the inhalation. Imagine an open channel from the crown of the head to the heart; then as you are inhaling, sense or imagine the breath/prana flowing from above the head downward through that channel and into the area of the heart.

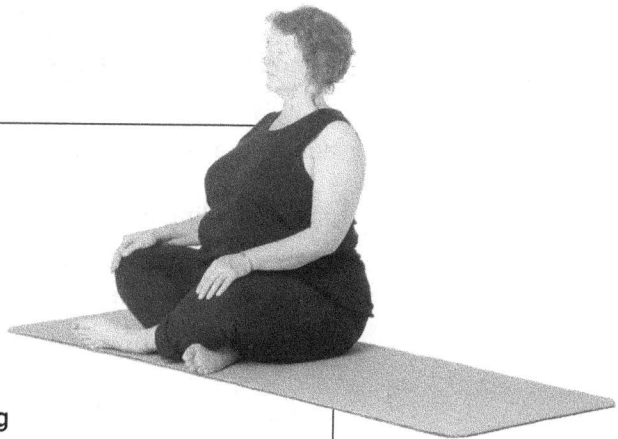

Awakening Prana

▼ Take a comfortable seated position.

▼ Sit quietly for a minute or so
to let your body and breath settle.

▼ Expand your exhalation slightly, keeping
it natural and comfortable.

▼ As you inhale, imagine/sense the flow of prana
like a stream of sunlight entering through the crown of your
head and flowing through the head and neck and
into the area of the heart.

▼ Give some attention to releasing muscular restriction through
the temples, jaw and neck.

▼ Repeat for 5 breaths and rest for 3 breaths.

▼ Do 5 rounds. Each round is 5 prana-awakening
inhalations followed by 3 resting breaths.

▼ Rest for a minute or so, seated or in **Savasana**.

Apana

Apana flows downward and outward. Starting at the lower back, apana flows down through the pelvis, the legs, the feet and into the earth. Apana is the energetic root connecting us to the planet.

Vital apana gives our body strength and stability. It is through vital apana that we can connect to and absorb earth energy. When we are well-connected to the earth through healthy apana we are grounded both physically and emotionally.

If we lack the support of apana, we will unconsciously compensate for this lack by gripping the muscles of our legs, pelvis and lower abdomen. Gripping in this way does give us some stability, but at the cost of losing vitality, mobility and responsiveness through the whole body. Just like a good root system allows a tree to move in the wind without breaking, healthy apana gives us mobility and ease through the hips, knees, ankles and feet, as well as freedom in the upper body.

The grounding energy of apana helps us to feel safe in our body and in life. It gives us a sense of quiet confidence. Apana supports us in being present to the moment and awakens in us a cellular knowing that we belong to the earth. Apana has an important stabilizing effect on the other four pranas.

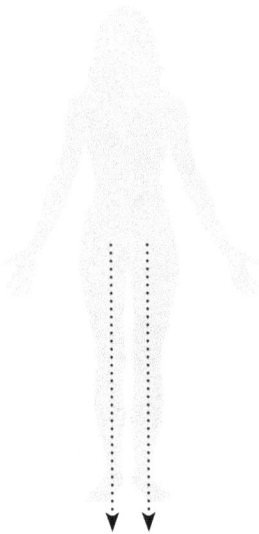

Apana is the energetic root connecting us to the planet.

Apana is the energetic communication between the torso and the legs. Good communication between the torso and legs is the basis of coordination between the upper and lower body. Lower back pain is frequently related to a lack of good communication between the legs and the torso. The psoas muscle, which is a deep muscle connecting the lower back to the legs, is a physical expression of this communication. An image of the psoas can be used as an inspiration for cultivating apana. It is particularly important in asana to tune into apana when we are focused on developing strength.

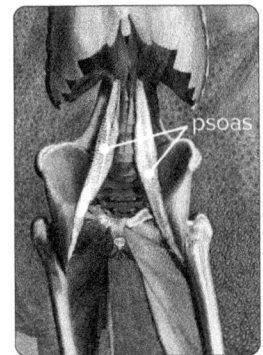

psoas

BERNARD SIEGRFRIED ALBINUS

Symptoms of imbalanced apana include menstruation difficulties, urination and defecation issues and sexual problems. Apana is also the energetic support for giving birth. It is worthwhile to cultivate apana if you would like to improve any of these functions.

Tension through the sacrum, tailbone, sitz bones, lower back and pelvic floor can restrict apana's flow. Doing asana with a focus on stimulating, balancing and releasing tension from these areas is an important contribution to awakening healthy apana.

We can awaken apana in asana by directing the exhalation through the pelvis and legs and into the ground. It can help to imagine these areas of the body as being empty and our exhalations flowing as if in one unbroken stream from the lower back, through the feet and into the earth. Standing and balance poses are good choices for working with apana.

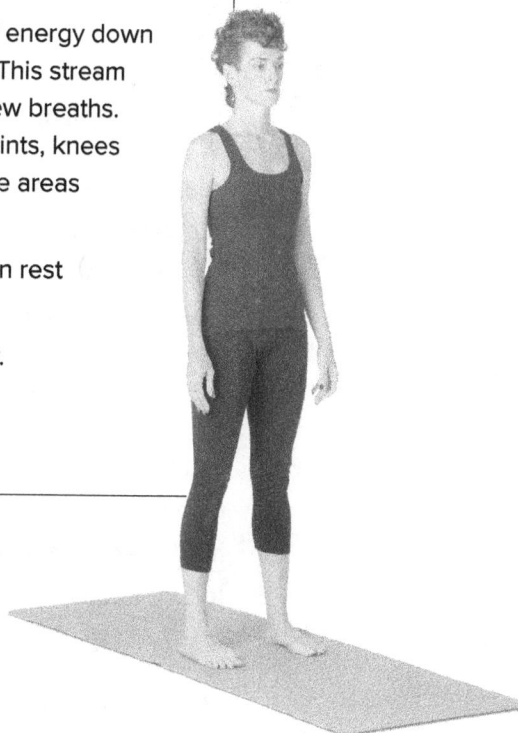

Awakening Apana

▼ Come into a **Mountain** pose with feet 6 to 8 inches apart so your body has an easy stability.

▼ Stand quietly for a minute connecting to the sensation of your breathing.

▼ Slightly increase the size of your inhalation.

▼ Exhale as if the breath is flowing like a stream of energy down through the pelvis, legs, feet and into the earth. This stream does not have to reach the ground on the first few breaths. Notice the breath/energy flow through the hip joints, knees and ankles since the flow of apana through these areas may be restricted.

▼ Breathe with apana in this way for 5 breaths, then rest for 3 breaths or until your system is quiet.

▼ Repeat 5 rounds of awakening apana in this way.

▼ Take a rest in **Savasana**.

Udana

UDANA

- Up and Out
- Diaphragm/Heart to Crown
- Balanced by Prana

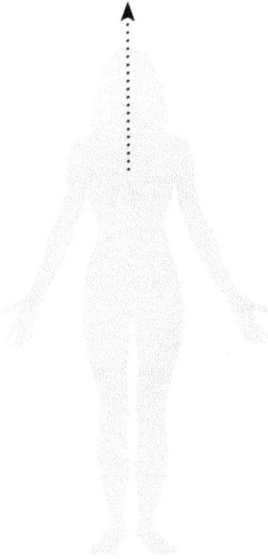

Udana is the upward and outward flow of prana. From the diaphragm and heart, udana flows upward through the chest, neck and head, exiting out through the crown of the head.

A buoyant chest, an uplifted heart and a vital upper spine all rely on healthy udana. Udana energetically supports joy, standing tall, and holding our head high. Exhaling through the crown of our head during asana is a good starting place for connecting to and awakening udana.

Exhaling, speaking and singing are functions of udana. It is with the help of vital udana that we are able to communicate clearly and speak confidently.

Udana also serves as our energetic connection to the universe and as such is support for getting in touch with more subtle levels of awareness.

If we are feeling heavy, depressed or blocked in any way, awakening udana can open and lighten us. If we are one of those people who has difficulty getting out of bed in the morning, stimulating udana can help us to wake up and get ourselves going.

Symptoms of imbalanced udana include trying to do too many things at once, problems with short-term memory and constantly feeling that we don't have enough time. Blocked udana can also cause headaches.

Udana serves as our energetic connection to the universe and ... is our energetic support for getting in touch with more subtle levels of awareness.

Udana and prana have a particularly close relationship because they flow in opposite directions along the same pathway. If one of these pranic flows is weak, restricted or disturbed, there will be a related imbalance in the other. In addition to cultivating udana and prana individually it is important to cultivate them in relationship to each other since many of the body functions that are supported by one are also supported by the other.

Skillful use of the upper body requires a balanced interplay of stability and mobility. This balanced interplay is possible only when the chest, neck and head have good udanic and pranic support. Udana and prana are essential for upper body integrity and so are important to keep in mind when we are working with the upper body actions of asana and pranayama.

Clarity in both prana and udana are particularly important for preventing compression and collapse through the chest, neck and shoulders while

PRANA

doing inversions. Lacking this support, inversions can lead to injury. Prana and udana are also the energetic underpinning for the vital upper-body actions required in Hero Poses.

Udana together with prana underlie communication between the heart and mind. Good heart/head communication is an important aspect of the confidence we need to fully trust, open to and connect with life.

We can cultivate udana and prana in relationship to each other by: exhaling upward and outward from the heart through the crown of the head; then inhaling from above the crown inward and downward to the heart. We can explore this interplay between udana and prana in asana practice, as a seated breath practice or in savasana. It is beneficial to practice using all three of these options.

Singing and chanting are great for cultivating **udana and prana**.

Awakening Udana

- ▲ Take a comfortable seated position.
- ▲ Sit quietly for a minute or so to let your body and breath settle.
- ▲ Expand your inhalation slightly, keeping your breathing natural and comfortable.
- ▲ As you exhale, imagine/sense the flow of prana like a stream of energy flowing from the heart and moving upward and outward through the crown of the head. Repeat 5 times.
- ▲ Rest for 3 breaths or until your nervous system is quiet.
- ▲ Do 5 rounds, each round being 5 udana-awakening exhalations followed by 3 resting breaths.
- ▲ Rest in a seated position or in **Savasana**.

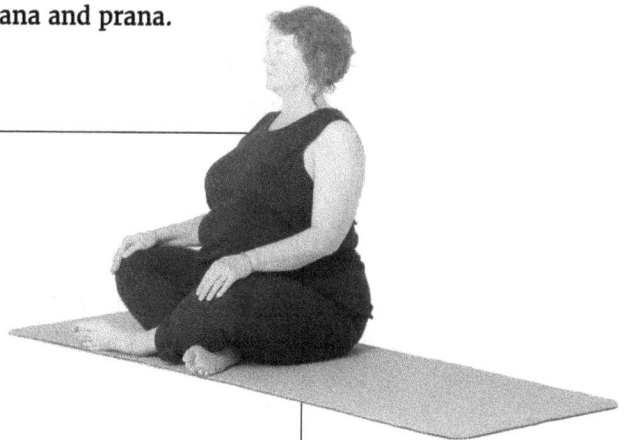

Vyana

Vyana is the outward-moving prana that starts in the heart and flows to and beyond the surface of the body. Vyana is the only pranic flow that moves through the whole body. We can think of it as our energetic circulatory system.

Blood flow is supported by and mirrors the movement of vyana. They are both centered in the heart and they both flow outward to the surface of our body, bathing every cell, tissue and organ along the way. While lymph circulation and nervous system flow do not so elegantly mirror vyana's movement, they are nevertheless both whole-body flows that are dependent on vyana for their health.

Vyana, along with the blood, lymph and nerve flow that it supports, are the cleansing, nourishing and communication systems of our body. Any area of our body in which any of these flows are restricted is prone to stagnation and vulnerable to poor health. Unobstructed, balanced flow in vyana and all of the systems it supports is one of the criteria of health.

Symptoms of imbalanced vyana include circulatory problems, which can express in a multitude of problems such as cold hands and feet and stagnation throughout the body. Other symptoms include heart problems and impaired reflexes.

Vyana is expansive, comprehensive and inclusive. It is the energy of our wholeness. Whole-body awareness, whole-body coordination and whole-self actions are expressions of vyana. Vyana is a valuable focus when working with expansive poses or when reintegrating parts of the body that have been injured. Problems in the periphery of our body such as cold hands and feet or peripheral neuropathy can also be helped by working with vyana.

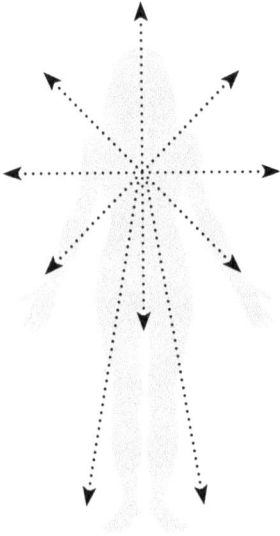

We can think of vyana as our energetic circulatory system.

In working with whole-body awareness, we are cultivating vyana. The reverse is also true. When we use the breath to awaken vyana, we are cultivating the foundation of whole-body awareness.

As the life energy flowing from the center to the periphery of our body, vyana is our energetic support for moving into and connecting with the people and life around us. If we teach or are in any other way responsible

PRANA

for communicating to groups of people, well-developed vyana helps us to fulfill those responsibilities without becoming depleted.

Openness, generosity and fearlessness are supported by vyana's outward-moving energy. So too is expressing ourselves, cooperating with others and influencing our communities. Vyana also underlies confidence and self-acceptance.

Physically, vyana, and all the dynamics it supports, lets us fully and generously extend through our arms, legs and spine in Hero poses, backbends and arm balances. Any expansive action, whether physical or emotional, is easier and more effective with the support of vyana.

The outward flow of vyana and the inward flow of samana balance each other. Each also serves as a basis for the other. Activating vyana creates an energetic aliveness in us that helps to stimulate samana, and vitalizing samana creates in us a vital center that serves as an energetic springboard for vyana.

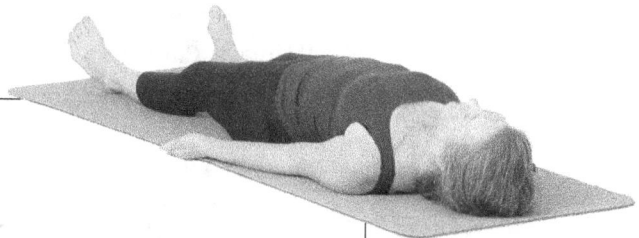

Awakening Vyana

* Lie on your back with legs extended. If needed, use supports to make yourself comfortable.

* Rest quietly for a minute or so to let your body and breath settle.

* Expand your inhalation slightly while keeping it natural and comfortable.

* As you exhale imagine/sense the flow of vyana as an outflow of energy, light or breath emerging from the heart and flowing in all directions through every cell of your body and slightly beyond the surface of the skin.

* Do this for 5 exhalations, then rest for 3 breaths.

* Do 5 rounds. Each round being 5 udana-awakening exhalations followed by 3 resting breaths.

* Rest.

Samana

Samana is centered in the navel region and is our inward-moving prana. Samana gathers, consolidates and concentrates. Its primary role in the body is in digestion. Poor or unreliable digestion and a irregular appetite are signs of disturbed samana.

Water spiraling down a drain is suggestive of the inward-drawing spiral action of samana. Just as a slow drain lacks a vital downward spiral and so the sink does not drain effectively, samana that is lacking in vitality is not able to support good digestion.

Strong digestion and good assimilation need healthy samana. Samana's spiral action underlies digestive power and samana's drawing action underlies the absorption of nutrients. Strengthening samana is an important practice for anyone wanting to improve their digestion.

The belly is an area of the body that people often want to change. Sometimes we want this change for digestive health reasons and sometimes for reasons of self-image. Cultivating samana improves digestion and it also provides a foundation for integrated strengthening of the entire abdomen.

Samana helps to prevent and resolve lower back pain by creating a cohesive relationship between the muscles of the abdomen and the muscles of the back. Abdominal muscles that are strengthened with the support of healthy samana are well organized, responsive and vital.

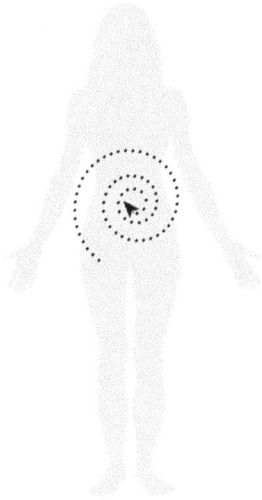

Strengthening samana is an important practice for anyone wanting to improve their digestion.

Abdominal muscles that are strengthened without samanic support lack aliveness. These muscles can be strong but they tend to be hard and unpliable and so do not work well together with the lower-back muscles. Abdominal strength that has been developed without samana can actually *cause* lower back pain.

A lack of healthy samana contributes to both abdominal tension and abdominal collapse. Abdominal collapse is a lack of vital samana, while excess abdominal tension is often a compensation for the lack of vital samana. Awakened samana integrates the abdominal muscles, which supports both the release of abdominal tension and the development of responsive abdominal strength.

Samana creates safety in backbends in a couple of important ways. The gathering, centering and toning effect of samana vitalizes the navel region and in doing so integrates the actions of the upper and lower body. And, as mentioned, samana protects the lower back by supporting muscular and functional integration between the abdomen and lower back.

As the pranic flow in the center of the body, well-developed samana anchors our entire pranic system. As such, samana is one of our best resources for staying centered. In addition to its value in yoga practices, the integrating action of awakened samana also helps us to sit comfortably, concentrate on a task and to stay focused as we move through our day.

Twists are good for stimulating samana. Samana plays a key role in maintaining equilibrium which makes balance poses and inversions valuable for exploring samana. Agni Sara* and Uddiyana Bandha* are powerful samana-stimulating practices but they have important contraindications and so should be learned from a teacher.

Vyana and samana are closely related and so in addition to cultivating them individually, it is important to spend some time working with them in relationship to each other.

Awakening Samana

- ◎ Come into **Child's Pose** using any supports you need to be comfortable.
- ◎ Take a minute or so to settle into the pose and become aware of your breathing.
- ◎ Expand your inhalation slightly, keeping your breathing natural and comfortable.
- ◎ As you exhale, feel a muscular activation around the navel and imagine/sense samana as an inward-spiraling energy that moves toward the spine.
- ◎ Repeat for 5 breaths, then rest for 2 or 3 breaths.
- ◎ Do 5 rounds — each round being 5 samana-awakening exhalations followed by 3 resting breaths.
- ◎ Rest in **Child's Pose** or **Savasana**.

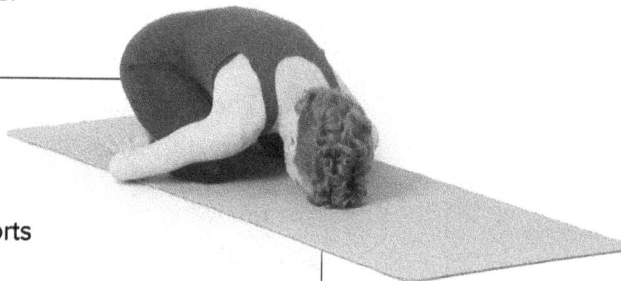

see Appendix, page 230

Cultivating the Five Pranas in Pairs

The following practices use natural, easy breathing with a slightly elongated inhalation and/or exhalation. As you work with the pranas, be aware of any area in your body where the pranic flow becomes thin, unclear, blocked or moves in the wrong direction. Let your awareness rest gently on this area as an invitation for the flow to improve. Resist any impulse to use effort for opening the flow.

You can explore the pranas either sitting or lying. Each position has its benefits so it is good to use both. Whichever position you choose, take a few minutes to become comfortable. Let your awareness rest on the movement of your breathing and wait for your body to become quiet and at ease. The more internally quiet you are, the greater will be your sensitivity to the breath/prana.

The following practices use natural, easy breathing (with a slightly elongated inhalation and/or exhalation) to explore cultivating pranas in pairs.

The following pranic pairs are just examples. There are many pairs you can create with the five pranas and all are valuable to explore. Once you become familiar with the basic idea of this practice you can explore pranic interplays that directly relate to specific asanas or areas of your body in which you are interested. The last exploration uses three pranas to introduce you to that possibility.

If you don't have time to explore all of the pranas at once, chose pranas that are related to an area of your body that you are interested in supporting.

PRANA

Prana & Udana

- Settle into a comfortable seated or lying position.

- As you inhale, imagine/sense prana flowing into the body through the crown of head, and descending into the area of the heart.

- As you exhale, imagine/sense udana flowing upward from the heart, through the neck and head, and out through the crown of the head. Keep your neck, jaw, scalp, temples and lips relaxed. Repeat for 7 - 10 breaths.

- Rest for a minute with a relaxed open awareness.

- Repeat the cycle 1 or 2 times.

- Rest as long as you like, noticing any awakening in prana and udana.

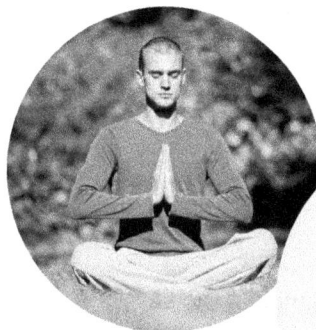

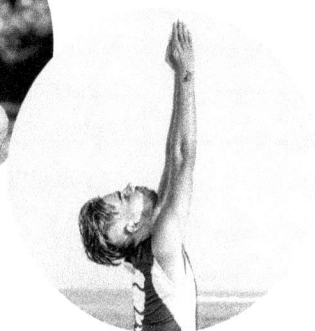

PRANA
through crown of head to heart

UDANA
from heart out crown of head

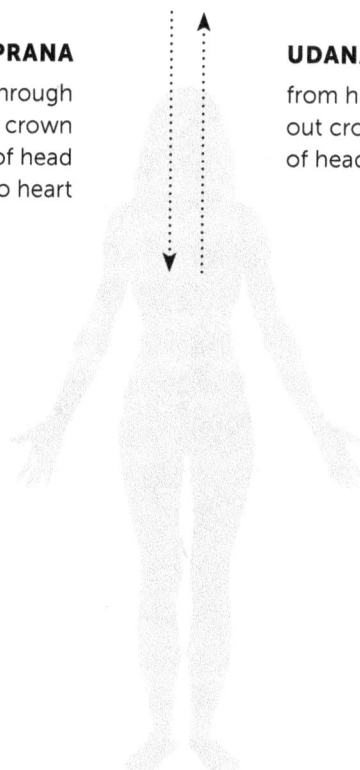

Prana & Apana

🌿 Settle into a comfortable seated or lying position.

🌿 As you inhale, imagine/sense prana entering the body through the crown of the head and flowing downward into the area of the heart.

🌿 As you exhale, sense/imagine apana flowing down through the pelvis and legs and into the earth. Repeat for 7 - 10 breaths.

🌿 Rest for a minute with a relaxed open awareness.

🌿 Repeat the cycle 1 or 2 times.

🌿 Rest with open awareness as long as you like, noticing any awakening in prana and apana.

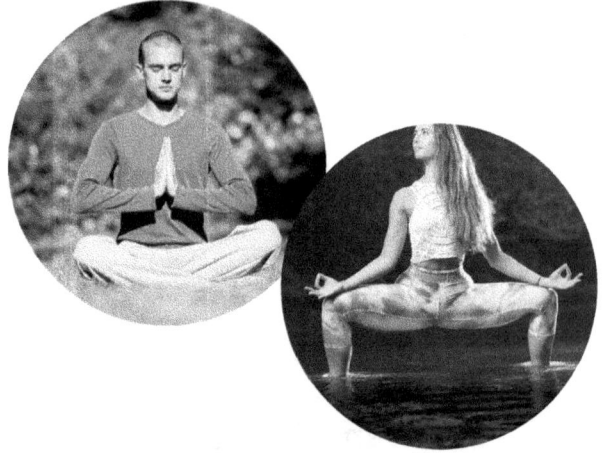

PRANA
through
crown
of head
to heart

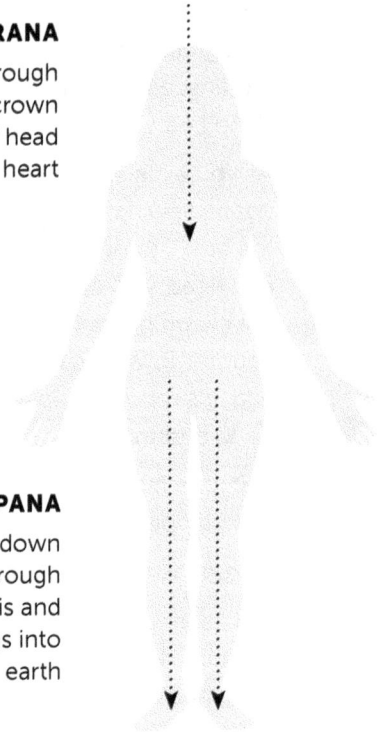

APANA
down
through
pelvis and
legs into
earth

PRANA

Prana & Vyana

🌿 Settle into a comfortable seated or lying position.

🌿 As you inhale, imagine/sense prana flowing into the body through the crown of head, and descending into the area of the heart.

🌿 As you exhale, sense/imagine vyana moving outward from the heart, flowing in all directions through the whole body to the skin and slightly beyond. Repeat for 7 - 10 breaths.

🌿 Rest for a minute with a relaxed open awareness.

🌿 Repeat the cycle 1 or 2 times.

🌿 Rest with open awareness as long as you like. Notice any awakening in prana and vyana.

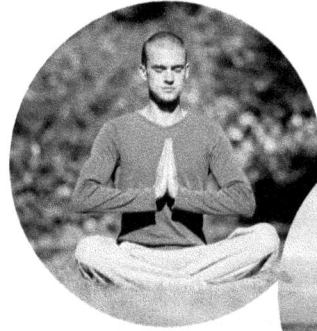

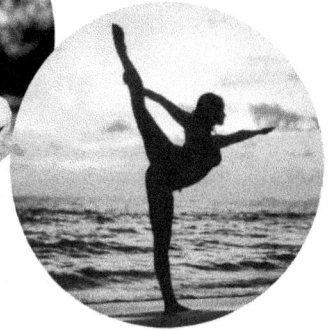

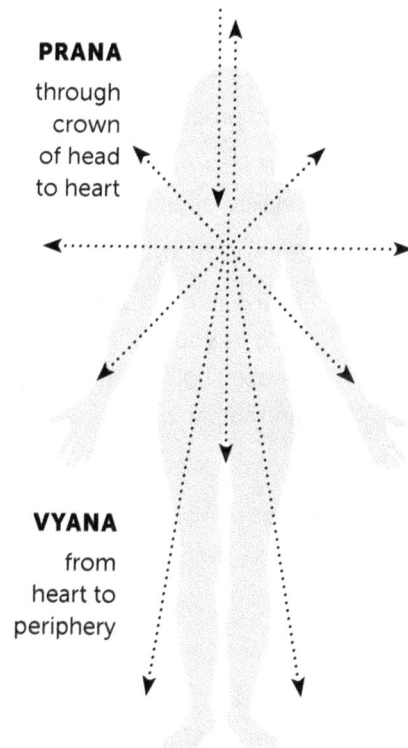

PRANA
through crown of head to heart

VYANA
from heart to periphery

Prana & Samana

- Settle into a comfortable seated or lying position.

- As you inhale, imagine/sense prana flowing into the body through the crown of head, and descending into the area of the heart.

- As you exhale, imagine/sense samana as an inward-spiraling energy moving from the navel toward the spine. Repeat for 7 - 10 breaths.

- Rest for a minute with a relaxed open awareness.

- Repeat the cycle 1 or 2 times.

- Rest with open awareness as long as you like, noticing any awakening in prana and samana.

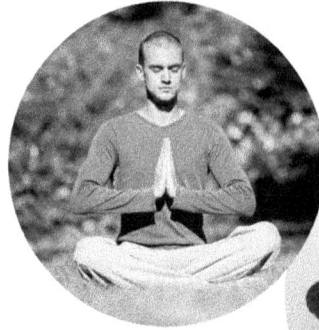

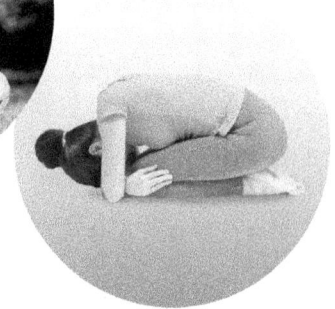

PRANA
through
crown of head
to heart

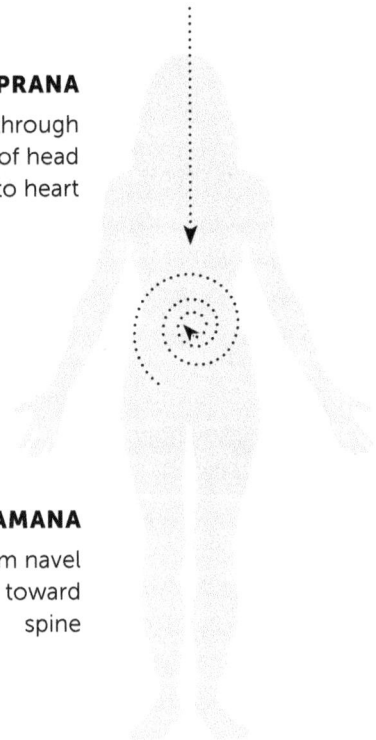

SAMANA
from navel
toward
spine

Vyana & Samana

- Settle into a comfortable seated or lying position.

- As you inhale, sense/imagine vyana moving outward from the heart, flowing through the whole body to and beyond the surface of the skin.

- As you exhale, imagine/sense samana as an inward-spiraling energy moving from the navel toward the spine. Repeat for 7 - 10 breaths.

- Rest with open awareness as long as you like, noticing any awakening in vyana and samana.

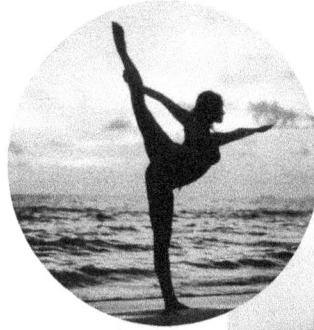

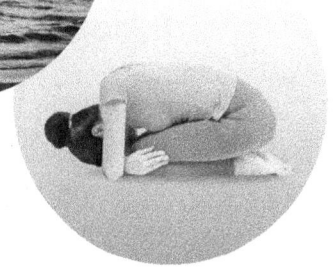

- Repeat the cycle 1 or 2 times.

- Rest in open awareness as long as you like, noticing any awakening in vyana and samana.

VYANA

from heart to periphery

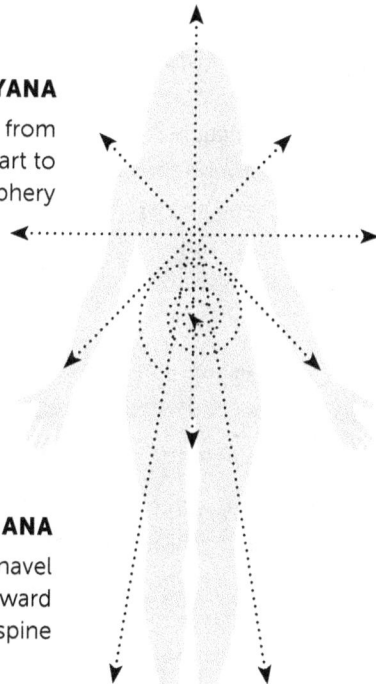

SAMANA

from navel toward spine

Prana & Apana & Udana

- ❧ Settle into a comfortable seated or lying position.

- ❧ As you inhale, sense/imagine prana flowing into your body through the crown of your head, moving downward to the area of the heart.

- ❧ As you exhale, sense/imagine apana and udana flowing out of the body equally and simultaneously in their directions — udana out through the crown of your head and apana down through your pelvis and legs and into the ground. Repeat for 5 breaths.

- ❧ Rest for a minute with a relaxed open awareness.

- ❧ Repeat the cycle 1 or 2 times.

- ❧ Rest with open awareness as long as you like, noticing any awakening in prana, apana and udana.

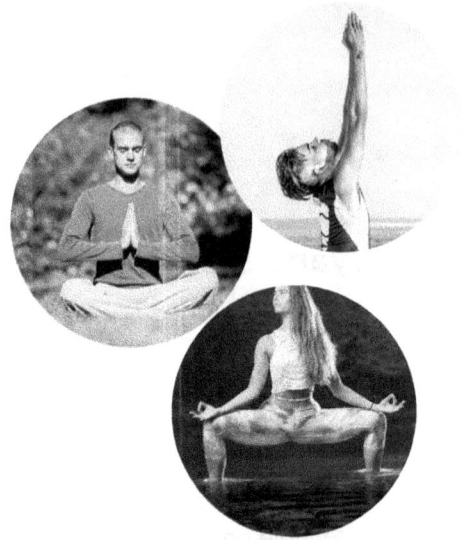

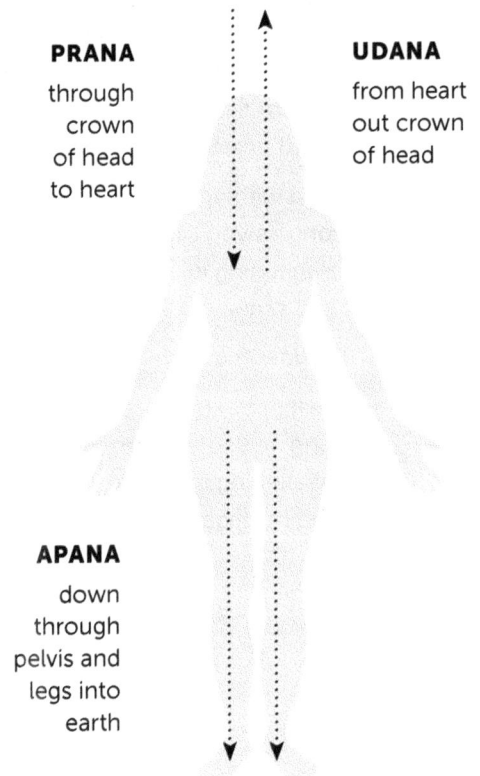

PRANA
through
crown
of head
to heart

UDANA
from heart
out crown
of head

APANA
down
through
pelvis and
legs into
earth

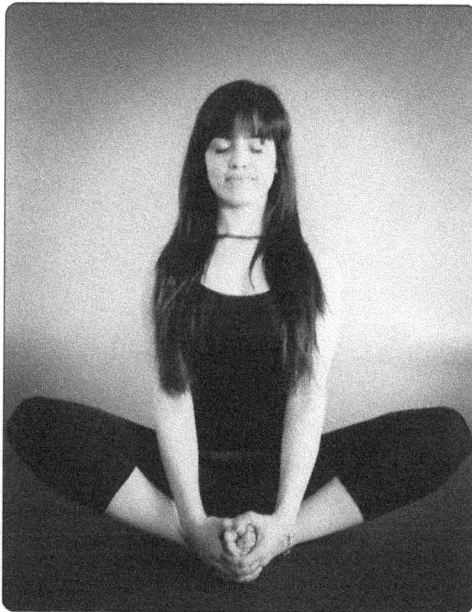

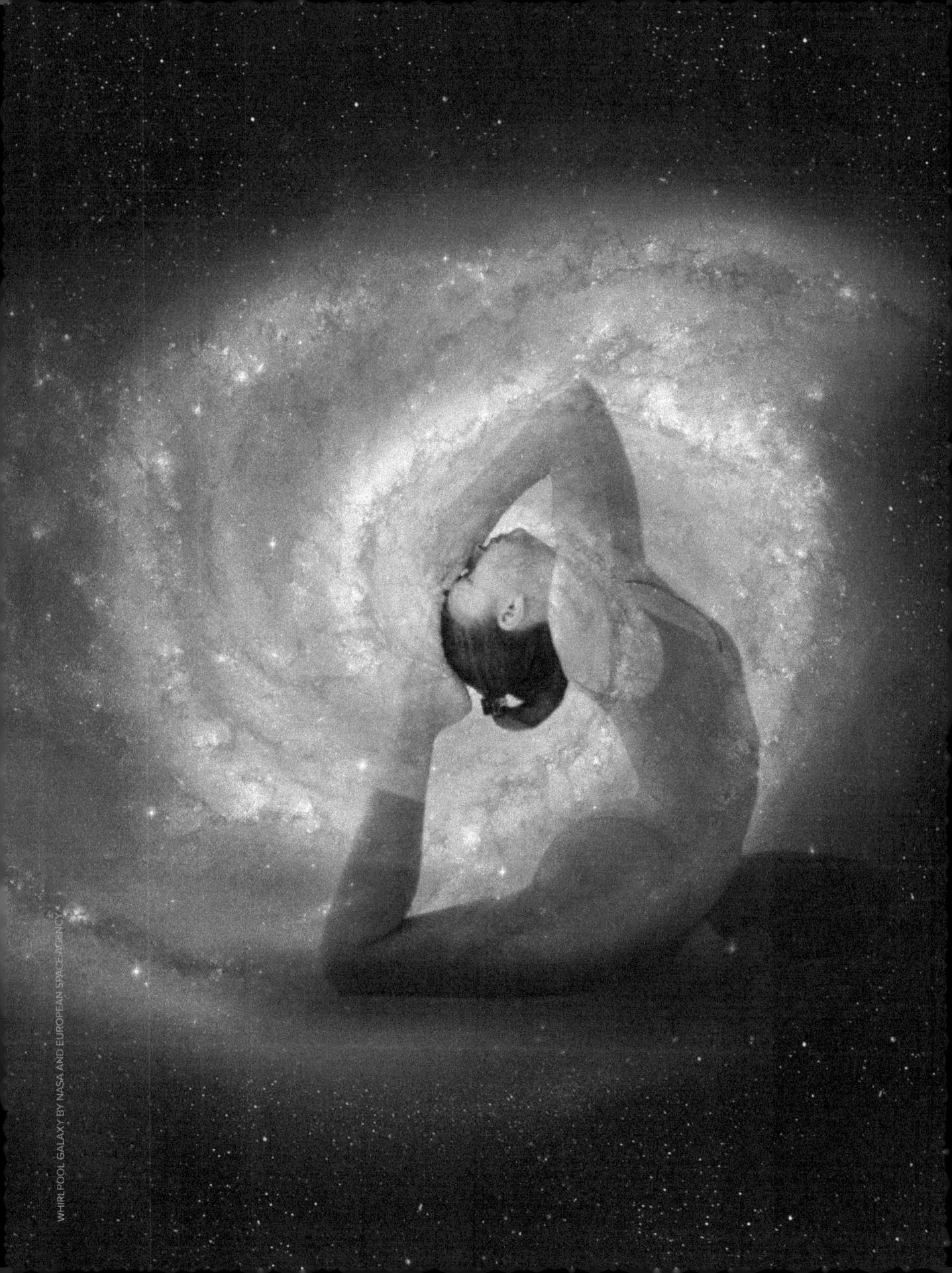

Part TWO

Creating
Ayurvedically Inspired
Yoga Practices

Introduction to the Practice Section

This section is organized as a 3-level approach to developing skill in using yoga practice for doshic balancing. These practices are designed for cultivating self-awareness through an Ayurvedic lens. Approaching the practices as meditation or as a somatic inquiry will yield the best results.

1st Level: Practice Focuses
Way of using attention to influence the effects of asana.

2nd Level: Practice Seeds
Options for increasing the dosha-balancing effect of any yoga practice.

3rd Level: Practice Sequences
Structured yoga practices for dosha-balancing.

Practice Focuses

Focuses describe different ways of using your attention in asana. Working with the Focuses is a means of both cultivating somatic awareness and of influencing the effect of a practice. Focuses can be used to address specific needs or interests. **Three types of Focuses are offered:**

> ≈ **Physical**   ≈ **Breath/Energetic**   ≈ **Mental/Emotional**

The Focuses are used as part of the dosha-balancing practices in this book, but Focuses on their own are not dosha-specific. They can be used for expanding the possibilities of any asana practice with or without an Ayurvedic intention. The description of each Focus includes one example of how it can be applied to dosha balancing.

Practice Seeds

Seeds are dosha-balancing principles organized as single points. They are designed to be integrated into a regular yoga practice. You can include one or many Seeds depending on your interests and needs. Giving a little attention to one or two Seeds during a practice slightly increases its dosha-balancing effect. If you want to create a stronger dosha-balancing effect, simply use more Seeds or stay attentive to one Seed throughout a whole practice.

Working with the Seeds gives you insight into how any practice can be used for dosha balancing. Seeds allow you to explore Ayurveda and yoga together at a relaxed pace within the comfort of a familiar practice. **Seeds are organized as:**

~ **Physical**   ~ **Breath/Energetic**   ~ **Mental/Emotional**

Practice Sequences

Sequences are yoga practices that are structured for dosha balancing. They are composed primarily of asanas that lend themselves well to balancing a specific dosha. A few breathing and meditation practices are also included. Focuses and Seeds are added to these sequences to increase their dosha-balancing effect. The combination of dosha-balancing asanas, Focuses and Seeds creates a strong dosha-balancing practice.

In addition to balancing doshas, exploring these practices gives you a good foundation for understanding how to be creative in developing your own Ayurvedically inspired yoga practices.

These three levels of practice are organized in this section as follows:

Table of Practices

The following is a complete list of practices that appear in this second section of the book.

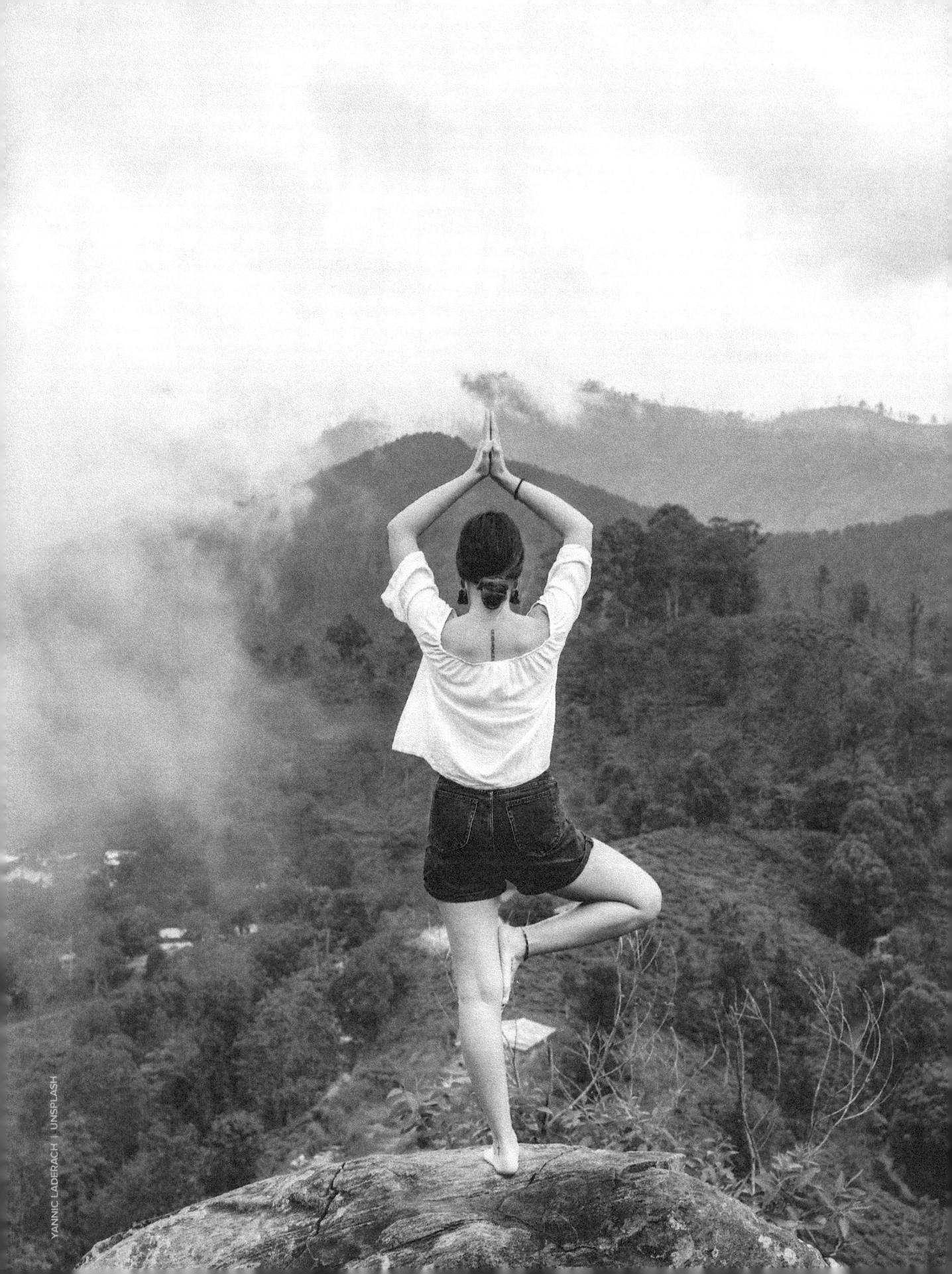

Focuses for Yoga Asana

Every asana has benefits created by how its shape stimulates our body. These benefits can be increased, modified or changed significantly by bringing different focuses and intentions to the asana during practice. A single asana can give us a wide range of benefits if we know different ways to focus and bring intention to it. The more options we have for working with asanas, the more skillfully we can meet our changing needs. Recognizing and meeting our changing needs is a primary dictate of Ayurveda.

The Focuses outlined in this chapter have two purposes: one is to cultivate different ways of being self-aware while doing yoga (somatic awareness); the other is to learn a variety of ways of using attention in asana for purposes of doshic balancing.

The Focuses are organized under three types:

- **Physical**
- **Energetic**
- **Mental/Emotional.**

These focuses can be used individually or in combination. You can choose Focuses based on your needs and interests, or just work through them to explore their effects. Learning a variety of ways to focus an asana practice also helps keep our practice alive and interesting. You will learn more ways of applying these Focuses to a practice in the upcoming chapters on doshic balancing.

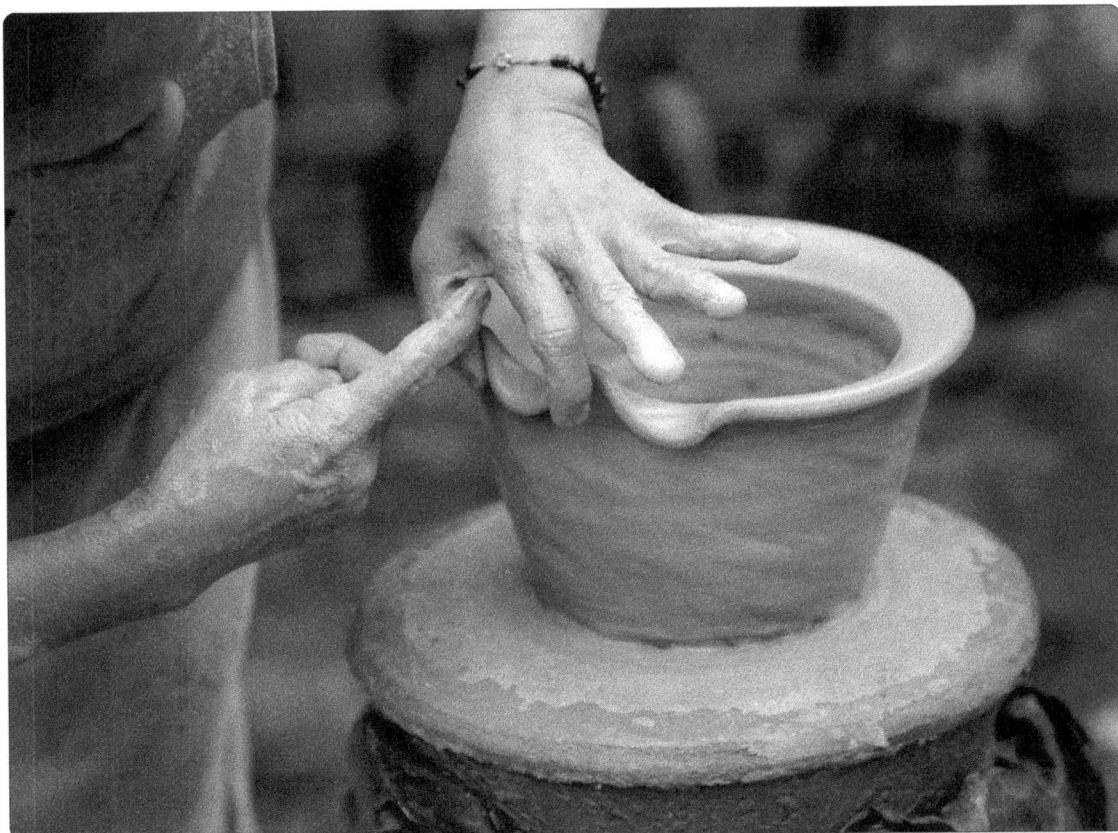

PHYSICAL FOCUSES

The Physical Focuses are:

- ☙ Form and Shape
- ☙ Joints and Bones
- ☙ Doshic Home Sites
- ☙ The Senses

Form & Shape

Just as a potter shapes clay into different forms, so too do we shape our body into asana forms. Muscular–skeletal alignments help us use our body in a more integrated way to make the asanas more effective. Alignments influence flow patterns in the blood, breath and prana, and allow us to focus an asana to massage specific internal organs. Alignments also encourage balanced muscular–skeletal action.

VATA	PITTA	KAPHA
Maintain awareness of the spine as your vertical midline and let it be a reference for balancing the two sides of the body.	Relax the lower back muscles away from the spine and soften around the heart.	Enliven the body by vitalizing the spine, feet and hands.

FOCUSES

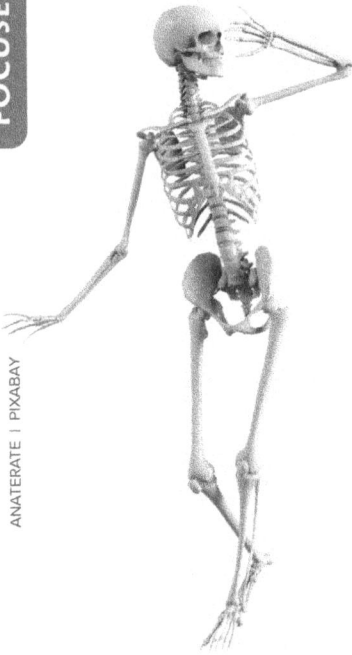

ANATERATE | PIXABAY

The Joints & Bones

There are a little over two hundred bones in our body and about half of those are in the hands and feet. The muscular system on the other hand has somewhere in the neighborhood of 700 muscles making it a more complex system.

The relative simplicity and clarity of the skeleton makes it an excellent focus for cultivating body alignment. The bones are an anti-gravity scaffolding around which our muscles organize. Aligning the joints and bones supports balanced, whole-body muscular action and encourages good placement of the organs.

VATA	PITTA	KAPHA
Cultivate physical stability by creating balanced action on the both sides of a joint. This helps counteract vata's tendency to excess mobility.	Cultivate a point of stillness in the center of the joints. This balances pitta's tendency to use excess effort.	Focus on creating space in the joints. This balances kapha's tendency to physical heaviness and density.

---❋---

Doshic Home Sites

ⓘ **Doshic Home Site** refresher on page 89.

Home sites are essential areas of focus in creating dosha-balancing practices. Vata's home site is the colon, pitta's is the stomach and kapha's is the lungs. Directing muscular actions in specific ways into these sites is an important part of developing Ayurvedically inspired yoga practices.

Squeezing, softening, massaging, stretching and mobilizing are some of the physical dynamics that asana can bring to a doshic site. These actions can be focused on an organ from different directions or angles for purposes of soothing, stimulating or mobilizing.

VATA
Colon

PITTA
Stomach
Liver
Small intestine

KAPHA
Lungs

VATA	PITTA	KAPHA
Use twisting asanas to create gentle but firm compressive and wringing actions in the torso on the level of the colon.	Soften and open space around the stomach, liver and small intestine in order to decompress these organs.	Use vigorous twists and backbends to activate the lungs.

The Five Senses

How we use our five senses powerfully influences our body. Muscular–skeletal balance or imbalance are wired together with our habits of using our senses. The senses are a powerful resource for cultivating asana because they give us an easy means of releasing unconscious tensions.

Simple actions such as relaxing the tongue or softening the eyes can reduce effort through the whole body and create a systemic quiet. Awareness of the muscles around the eyes, ears, nostrils and tongue can be used to monitor muscular tone through our body so we can recognize and release tension or activate underused muscle.

VATA

Open and enliven the inner ears as if listening to a leaf move in a quiet forest. Maintaining throughout a practice creates internal balance.

PITTA

Relax the muscles around the eyes, let the eyes soften and go into peripheral vision. Maintaining through a practice counteracts pitta's tendency to over-focus.

KAPHA

Dilate nostrils and wake up the tissues inside the nose as taking in the smell of a fresh, spring air. Maintain through a practice to enliven the breath and body.

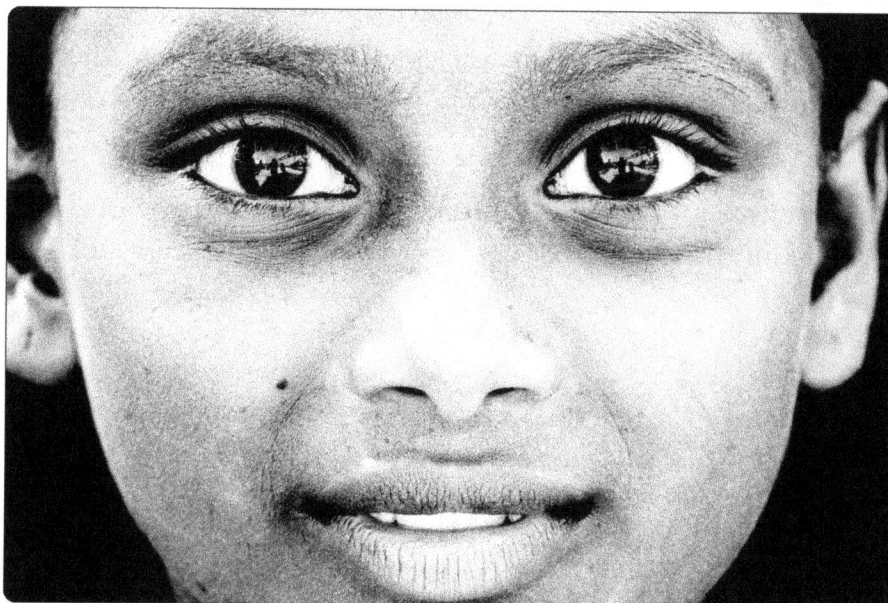

NEOSIAM 2020 I PEXELS

BREATH/ENERGETIC FOCUSES

Energy Focuses work with the subtle body. The subtle body is the energetic foundation of the physical body so clarifying the subtle body helps refine the physical body. In cultivating the subtle body our physical body becomes more responsive and sensitive.

"Yoga is ... the exploration and discovery of the subtle energies of life."

— Amit Ray

The Energetic Focuses are:
- ☞ The Breath
- ☞ The Five Pranas
- ☞ The Five Elements.

The Breath

Free, natural breathing is the best starting place for engaging the breath in asana. All asanas affect the breath through the demands they make on the muscles of respiration. Asana also affects our breathing by how it interacts with our personal habits of breathing. Cultivating free breathing in asana can be as simple as softening areas of tension or restriction in the body. Releasing of tension anywhere in the body encourages another degree of freedom in breathing.

Different styles of yoga use the breath differently. Any way of working with the breath is more effective when done on the foundation of relaxed, responsive muscles of respiration.

An easy way to use breathing for doshic balance in asana is to breathe as if the breath is flowing in and out of the body through the home site of a dosha.

ⓘ **Doshic Home Site** refresher on page 89.

VATA	PITTA	KAPHA
Cultivate a long, soft exhalation to help ground vata.	Breathe as if the breath is entering and leaving the body through the skin. This helps to soften the pitta tendency to over-heat.	Vitalize both the inhale and exhale to enliven the body and breath. This helps to balance kapha's tendency toward sluggishness.

The Five Pranas

The Five Pranas are one of the most effective and enjoyable ways of developing the energetic aspect of asana practice. The close relationship between breath and prana makes breathing the easiest access into engaging the pranas.

Start with awareness of the entire length of the exhalation, then merge the exhalation with the different flow patterns of the pranas. Initially you will be more aware of the breath itself but with a little time you will sense the flow of prana.

Start by clarifying the five pranas individually.

Five Pranas refresher, page 127.

VATA	PITTA	KAPHA
Cultivate **apana** to help tether vata's mobile nature (see sidebar).	Emphasize **vyana** to diffuse pitta's intensity.	Cultivate **udana** to lift kapha out of its tendency toward lethargy.

APANA

Down and out, lower abdomen, pelvis, legs

VYANA

Center to periphery, heart to surface

UDANA

Up and out, diaphragm/heart to crown

The Five Elements

Just as a dancer expresses different qualities in movement so too can we cultivate different elemental qualities in asana. Infusing asanas with elemental qualities is an effective way to balance doshas.

Elements refresher, page 38.

VATA	PITTA	KAPHA
Ground vata's lightness and mobility by contemplating the solid nature of earth and allowing the feeling of that solidity to permeate the entire body.	Engage water and earth's coolness to balance pitta's hot nature.	Stimulate the mobility of air and the heat of fire to counteract kapha's heaviness.

MENTAL/EMOTIONAL FOCUSES

Mental/Emotional Focuses gather the power of the mind and emotions behind a goal. A clear intention in the mind harnesses all of our energies in our body. An intention is not a demand or an expectation.

A Mental/Emotional Focus can be set in a brief moment at the beginning of a practice, reaffirmed periodically during the practice and then touched into again at the end. Or it can be held as a tone in the background of our awareness during the whole practice.

The Mental/Emotional Focuses are:
- Intention (Physical and Emotional)
- Imagery.

Intention

We always have an intention when doing a practice, even if it is not conscious. A conscious intention points our energies in a specific direction. An intention could be on healing an injury, resolving a chronic health problem, healing emotionally or growing spiritually. Whatever our Focus, articulating it clearly and simply to ourselves before starting our practice combines the power of the mind with the cultivation of the body.

Physical Intentions

VATA	PITTA	KAPHA
Create an intent to cultivate stillness in mind and body during asana to balance vata's tendency toward excess movement.	Have the intent to reduce effort in asana in order to counteract pitta's inclination to work harder than necessary.	Maintain a strong, clear focus to the details of an asana to counteract kapha's tendency toward dullness.

Emotional Intentions

VATA	PITTA	KAPHA
Let go of fear and trust life to balance vata's tendency to being fearful and anxious.	Let go of anger and invite contentment to counteract pitta's inclination toward heated emotions.	Let go of attachment and invite surrender to counteract kapha's tendency to hold on to things.

Imagery

Our brain thinks in pictures so imagery is a great resource for shaping our asana practice. If we are challenged by an asana, gazing at an image of someone doing it with ease allows us to experience their ease by osmosis.

Nature images can be wonderfully helpful for our practice, indeed the names of the asanas often provide us an image. For example, our Cobra pose can be enlivened by gazing at a photo of an upright cobra. Images can also help us access energies and qualities: an image of a tiger playing can help us connect to our inner power and energize our physical strength; birds in flight can inspire us to surrender and be carried by life; a mountain can inform us about stability and confidence.

VATA

Imagine lying comfortably on your belly on warm earth. Imagine an umbilical cord growing from your navel deep into the earth. Allow yourself to be nourished by earth energy coming through that cord and into your belly. This image grounds vata's airy nature.

PITTA

Imagine resting by a peaceful lake in evening under a radiant silvery moon. Let your body, mind and heart be soothed and cooled by the shimmering water and the soft glow of silver moonlight. This image balances pitta's fiery nature.

KAPHA

Imagine standing on the top of a mountain, gazing out over a vast landscape and feeling a breeze on your skin. Imagine your body and mind expanding to receive the landscape and breeze into yourself. Exploring this image as an inner experience brings spaciousness and mobility into kapha's dense nature.

These images can be engaged actively in asana or meditatively in Savasana.

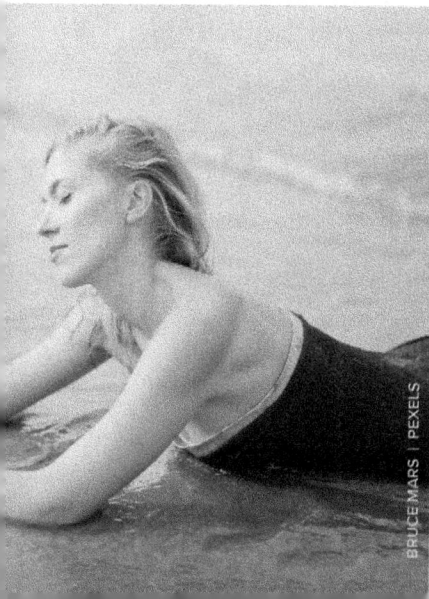

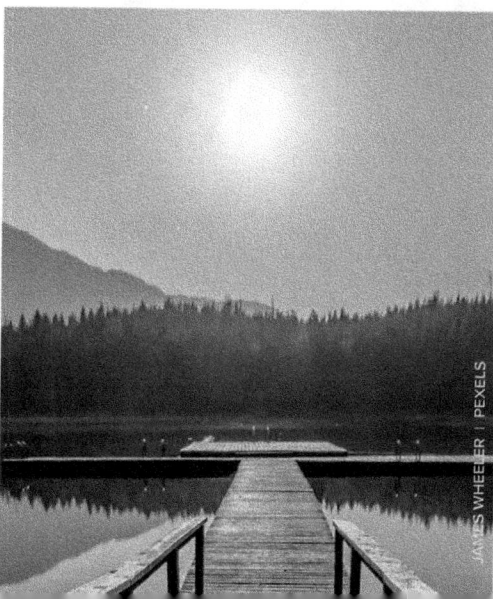

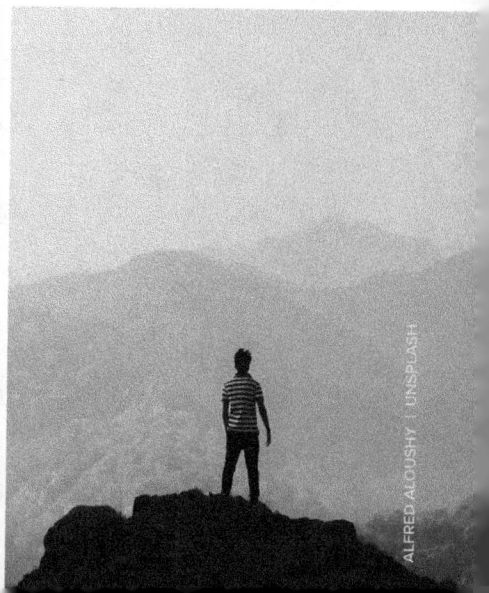

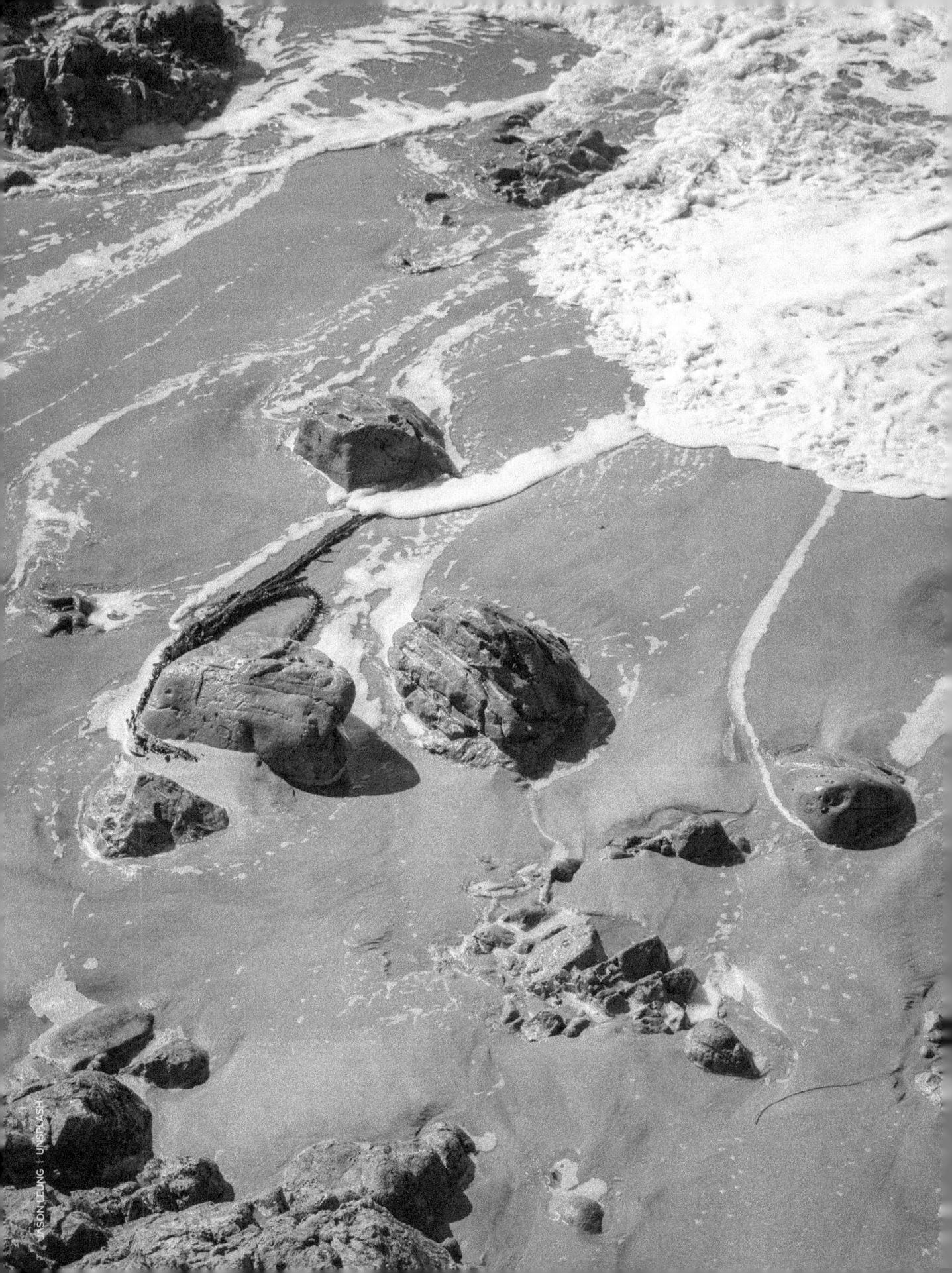

Vata-Balancing Practices – Controlling Wind

For thirteen years I lived across the street from the Caribbean Sea. On windy days the kite surfers would emerge. Watching them was one of my favorite pastimes. They strapped their feet to boards, tethered themselves to huge colorful kites with long reins, and then sat in the water. When they found just the right relationship to the wind, they were lifted upright and carried across the water on their wind-supported adventure.

Sometimes they would slow down so much it seemed surely that there was nowhere for them to go but down. Magically another wind would lift them up and carry them off in the other direction. As they gained speed, holding firm to their reins, they and their boards would become airborne and they would somersault through the air.

This is a glimpse of an experienced kite surfer. An inexperienced one creates a much less elegant picture.

The balanced tension between a kite surfer, his kite and the wind is an exquisite interplay of man and nature. Controlling vata is like kitesurfing. A kite surfer skillfully engages air in the form of wind, while a practitioner of yoga and Ayurveda skillfully engages air in the form of vata.

Vata is powerful and unpredictable and while controlling it is less dramatic than kitesurfing, regulating vata requires as much sensitivity and skill as sailboarding. Uncontrolled vata tosses us around in our lives in the same way that the wind dumps an inexperienced kite surfer into the water. Skillfully navigating vata is the foundation of our health and well-being.

Practice Seeds for Balancing Vata

Integrating one or more of the following vata-balancing Seeds into your asana practice boosts its vata-balancing effect. For a stronger effect, simply use more Seeds.

PHYSICAL SEEDS FOR BALANCING VATA

Doshic Home Site refresher on page 97.

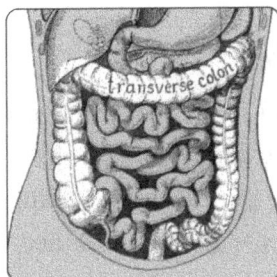
transverse colon

Attend to Vata Home Site

The colon is the home site of vata so directing the action of asana to massage, stimulate and balance the pelvis and lower abdomen is an important focus for vata balancing.

| Massage the colon through muscular actions, e.g., twists. | Create symmetry and stability in the pelvis to support proper structure and function of the colon. | Stimulate the colon through asanas that press the belly into the floor, e.g., cobra and bow. |

Align Joints

Vata people often have hypermobility and joint instability. Aligning and balancing the joints during asana provides stability. Joint balancing also creates a systemic quiet that soothes vata.

| Balance the muscular action on the outside and inside of the wrists, elbows, ankles and knees. | Stabilize the hip joints by an inward and slightly upward direction of pressure of the greater trochanter into the hip joint. | Cultivate a point of stillness in the center of the joints. Start with 2 joints and work up to 4. The shoulder and ankles are a good place to start. |

Connect to Earth

Vata's light and mobile nature needs grounding. When grounded, vata expresses as enthusiasm, creativity and playfulness. When ungrounded, vata expresses as anxiety, an inability to focus, and instability.

In standing poses yield the weight of your pelvis, sacrum and legs into the earth in order to more fully receive the uprising force of ground force.

Stabilize the legs by aligning the centers of the hip, knee and ankle joints.

Explore different points of contact of the feet on the floor to awaken the feet's potential for full receptivity to earth energy:
- between the big and 2nd toe;
- the 4 corners of the foot;
- the triangle created by the 2 corners of the balls of the feet and the centers of the heels.

Emphasize Symmetry & the Midline

Vata bodies tend to be asymmetrical which leads to structural and functional imbalances. Attending to physical symmetry in asana helps to counteract this tendency. It is important to remember that the goal is learning to use the body with more functional balance, not make our structure perfectly symmetrical. All bodies are and always will be asymmetrical to some degree.

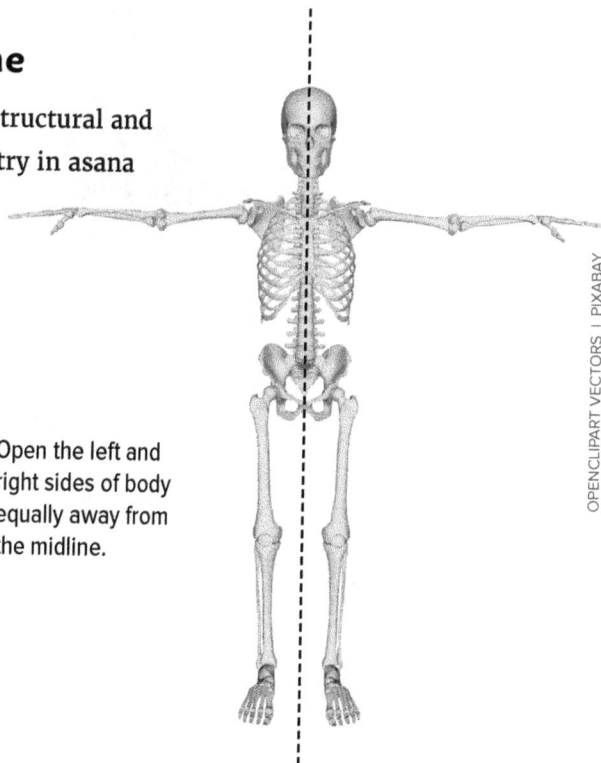

OPENCLIPART VECTORS | PIXABAY

Awaken and strengthen your sense of the body's vertical midline.

Use symmetrical poses to cultivate symmetrical action in your body, e.g., Mountain, Downward Facing Dog, Cobra, Child's Pose.

Open the left and right sides of body equally away from the midline.

Cultivate Strength & Endurance

Vata's energy and strength is variable. On any given day their response to the same stimuli can be very different, making it difficult to predict how they will respond to physical challenge. Slow, steady and incremental is the best approach for vatas in developing strength and endurance.

Gradually cultivate increased duration and steadiness in asana.	Build strength and endurance slowly and gently using a rhythm of alternating effort with rest.	Slow, meditative vinyasas are a good way for vata to develop endurance.

—※—

Engage the Senses

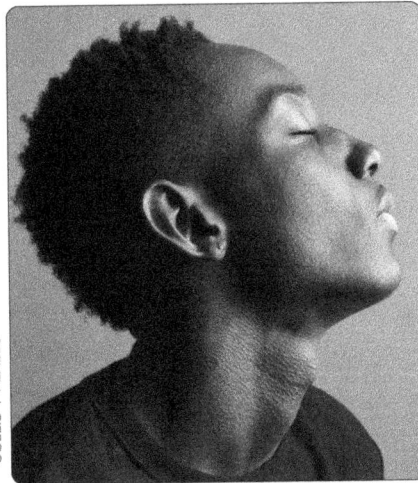

COLLIS | PEXELS

The potency of working with the senses makes them valuable for balancing all of the doshas, but especially for vata. Vata's sensitivity gives them easy access to the balancing possibilities of working with the senses. The skin and the ears are particularly good for vata balancing. The eyes are also useful.

Cultivate awareness of the surface of your skin as a soft, cushiony container for your whole body and feel it connecting to the space around you in asana.	*Perk up* your ears and listen with your whole body as if listening to the deep silence in a forest. You can also listen to the breath in this way.	Let your eyes rest softly in the sockets and descend downward toward the heart.

BREATH/ENERGETIC SEEDS
for BALANCING VATA

Breath

Vata's variable nature expresses as irregularity on many levels, including in breathing. Tethering and regulating the breath stabilizes vata.

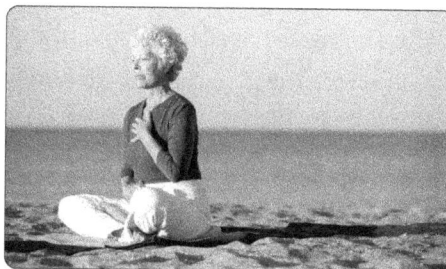

AMMENTORP | DREAMSTIME

Become aware of your lower back as a place from which to initiate breath.

Allow both lungs to fill equally and gently lengthen the exhalation.

Learn to relax momentarily in the pause at the end of the exhalation.

Prana

Of the 5 major directions of pranic flow in the body, apana is the most important for vata balancing. Samana and prana can also be helpful.

Strengthen **apana** by sensing your feet. Imagine/ sense roots growing deep in the earth from the entire bottom surface of your feet.

Balance **samana** by drawing prana inward toward the navel as you exhale.

Clarify **vyana** by creating an outward flow of prana from the heart as you inhale.

APANA
Down and out, lower abdomen, pelvis, legs

SAMANA
Periphery to center, inward belly spiral

VYANA
Center to periphery, heart to surface

Elements

Earth is the most valuable elemental energy for bringing solidity to vata's air and space nature.

Focus on stillness of body and mind during practice.

Cultivate the slow, steady pace of earth.

Give the body an experience of weight in Savasana by putting sand bags on the upper thighs and/or an eye bag over the eyes.

ℹ
Pranas
refresher on page 130.

Earth refresher on page 45.

MENTAL/EMOTIONAL SEEDS
for BALANCING VATA

These Practice Seeds can be used actively in asana or as a meditation. When using the Seeds in asana, the physical challenge should be reduced to allow for the attention needed to focus on the Seeds.

Intention

Release fear and anxiety on the exhalation.

Cultivate a trust of life on the inhalation.

Practice stillness of mind and body.

Imagery

In Savasana, imagine/sense yourself being covered with soft, warm sand.

In Savasana imagine floating in water and surrendering your body into that fluid support.

Resting on your stomach imagine growing an umbilical cord into the earth and taking in earth energy through that cord.

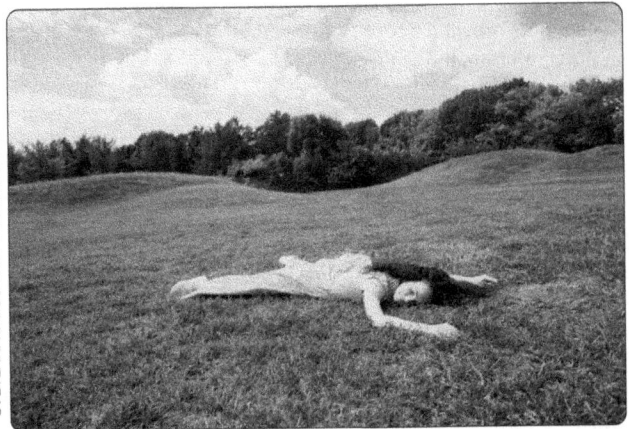

SVETLANA IAKUSHEVA | DREAMSTIME

Yoga allows you to find an inner peace that is not ruffled and riled by the endless stresses and struggles of life.

— B.K.S. Iyengar

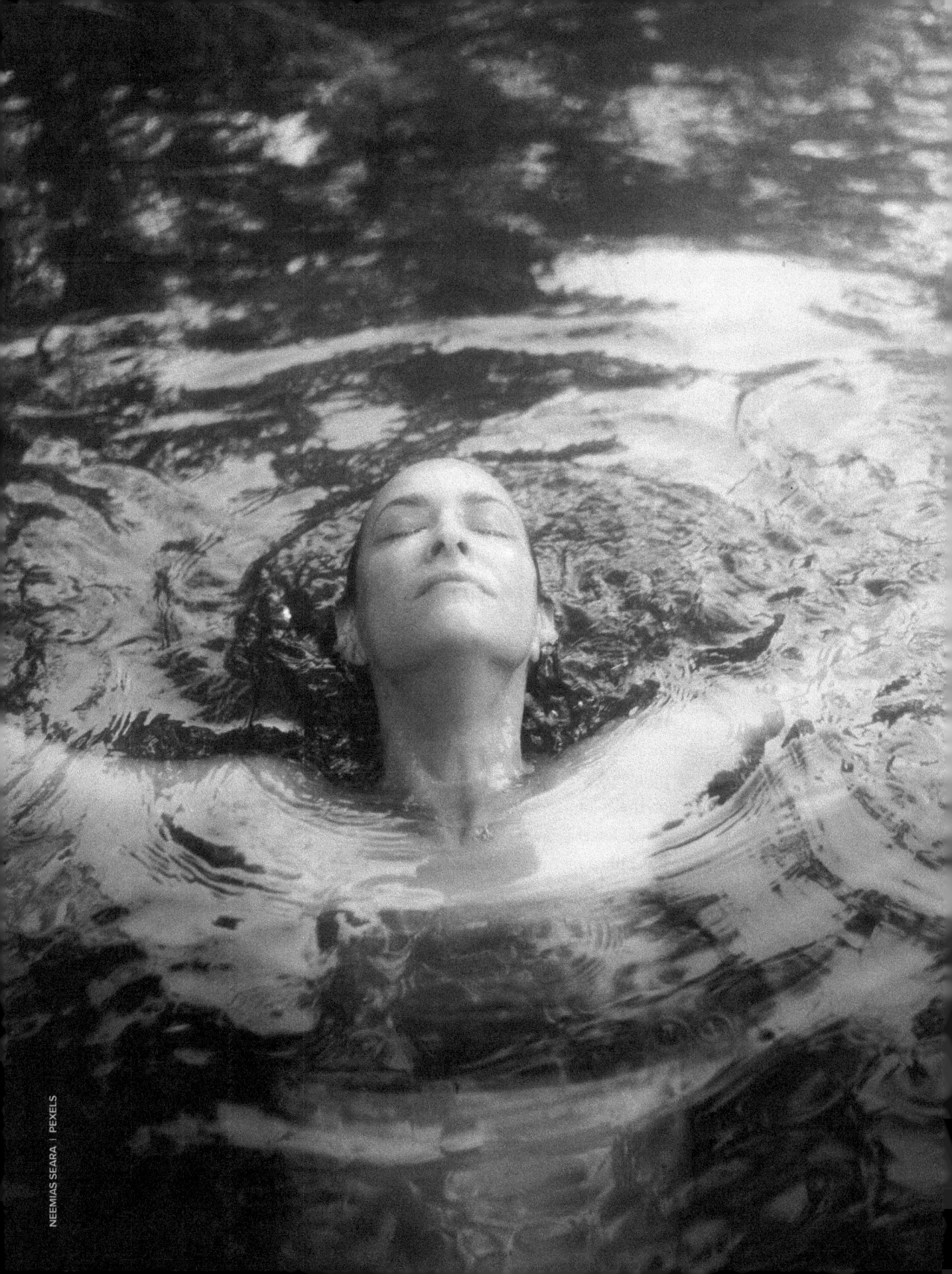

Practice Sequences for Balancing Vata

Home Site Practice for Vata

🕐 30 minutes

The goal of this practice is to get in touch with, massage and deeply relax the home site of vata. Use the image of the colon to refresh your memory about its shape and location. In working with the following asanas you can focus on the colon itself or on the whole lower belly. Either is fine, it is only a matter of preference.

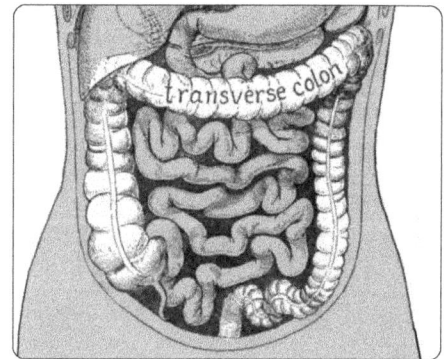

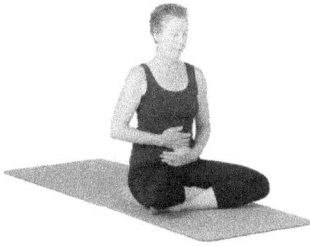

SITTING with HANDS on BELLY Sense the touch of your palms on your belly. Bring your awareness to the warmth of your hands and the movement of your breathing being aware of the colon as the home site of vata.

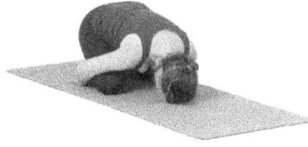

CHILD'S POSE Sense the movement of breath between the belly and thighs. Place a pillow between your belly and thighs if your body does not fold easily in Child's Pose.

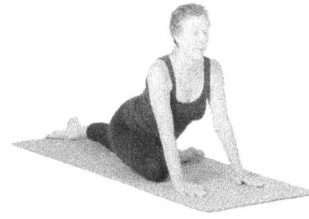

BABY PIGEON (both sides) Hold your awareness and breathe on the compression of the front-leg side of the abdomen and the stretch through the back-leg side of the abdomen.

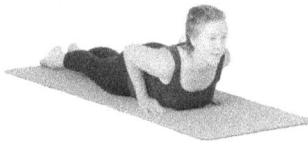

COBRA Breathe into the contact that the lower abdomen has with the floor and sense the stretch through the muscles and organs.

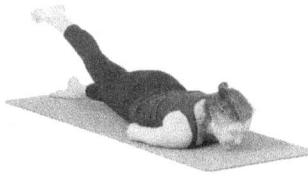

LOCUST (both sides) Make fists and press them into your abdomen in the area of the colon. Maintain the strength of your fists as you elongate and lift the left leg into the air. Breathe into the area of contact between your fists and your belly. Repeat with the right leg.

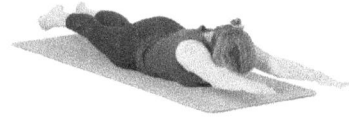

BOAT Hold your awareness and breathe in your lower abdomen. Sense and receive the pressure created by the abdomen's contact with the floor as you lift the arms, legs and head.

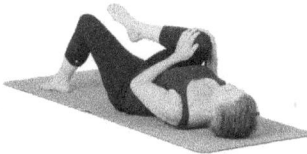

WIND RELIEVING POSE (both sides) Press your right thigh into the right side of your lower belly. Sense the contact between the thigh and lower belly and notice the increase in pressure on the inhalation and the decrease in pressure on the exhalation. Repeat on the left side. Place a towel or pillow between the thigh and belly if your thigh does not easily meet the belly.

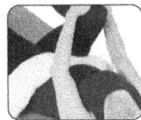

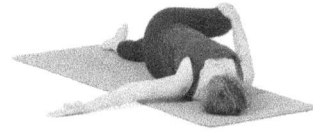

PASSIVE BENT KNEE TWIST (both sides) Start with right leg long and left knee bent. As you twist focus the spiral action of the twist into the right side of the lower abdomen. Repeat on the other side.

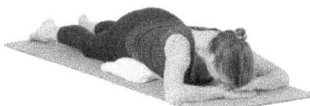

CROCODILE on a PILLOW Rest on your belly. Sense the movement of the belly pressing into the floor on the inhalation and moving away from the floor on the exhalation. Putting a folded towel under your belly can be useful. Start with ½ inch and experiment with different heights.

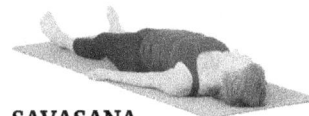

SAVASANA Rest.

Joints Practice: Align the Joints

🕐 40 minutes — for a 25 minute practice, omit asanas with an *

Aligning the joints creates physical stability and supports whole body integration. It also balances vata's tendency toward hypermobility and muscular skeletal imbalances.

To align a joint, simply balance the muscular action on opposite sides of the joint. You can use any two opposing sides. In ball and socket joints, such as are in the hips and shoulders, the pose that you are doing will help you know which two sides of the joint that it makes sense to use.

The following practice offers two sets of joints per asana to use as points of attention. Feel free to use one set of joints if two does not come easily to you. As you become more familiar with aligning the joints you can use as many joints as you are able to track.

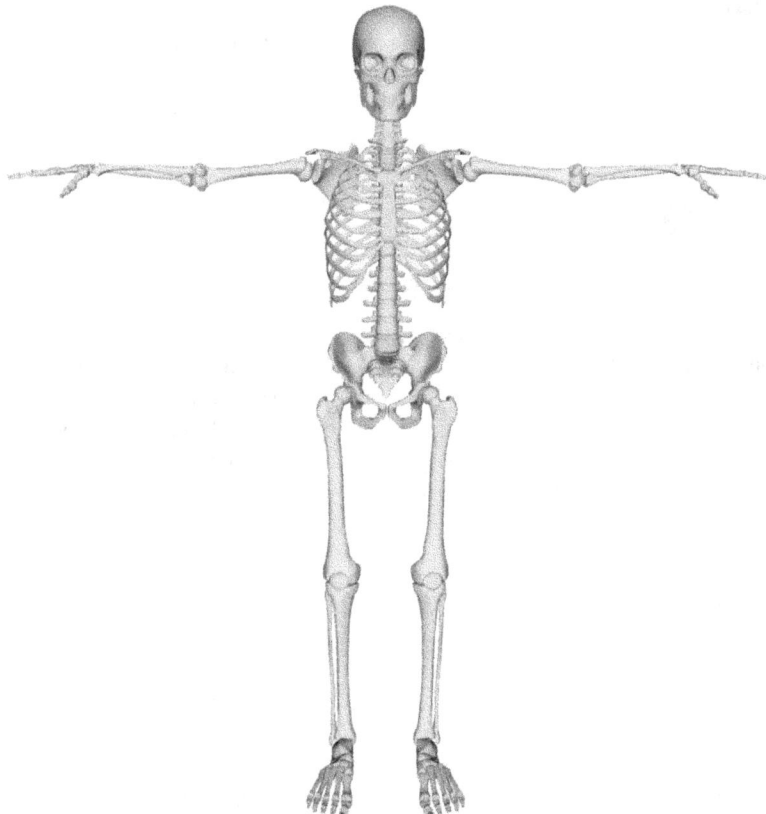

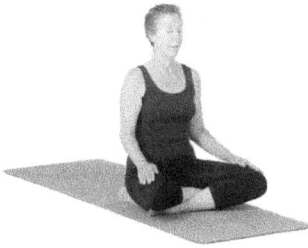

SEATED MEDITATION POSITION
Ankles and shoulders.

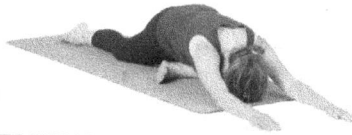

PIGEON LEGS (both sides)
Back leg knee
and front knee ankle.

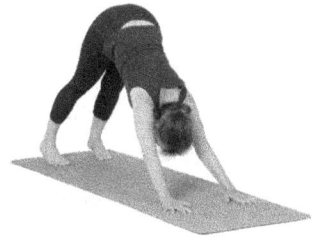

DOWNWARD DOG
Wrists and elbows.

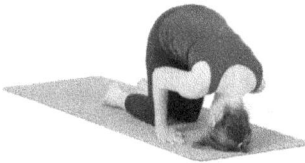

RABBIT
Shoulders and hips.

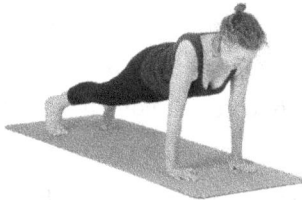

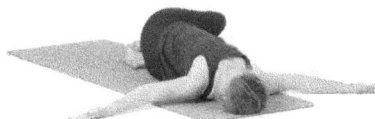

PLANK
Shoulders and ankles.

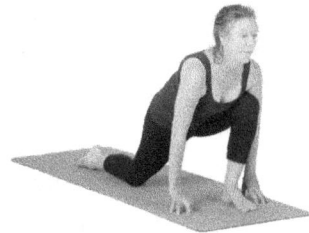

LUNGE (both sides)
Front knee and back ankle.

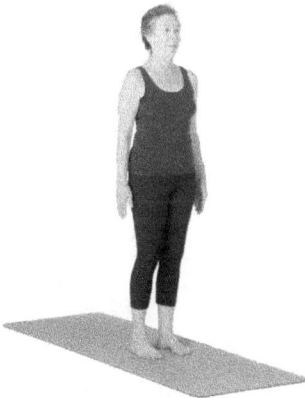

* MOUNTAIN
Ankles and knees.

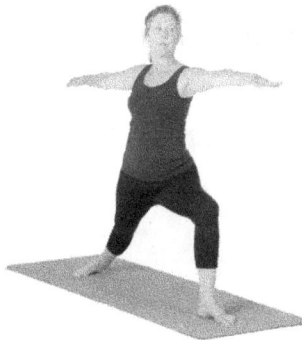

* HERO II (both sides)
Back knee and front ankle.

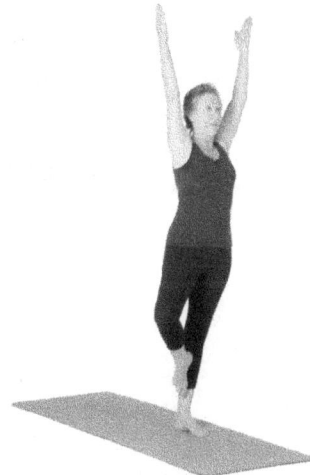

* TREE (both sides)
Standing leg hip and
lifted knee ankle.

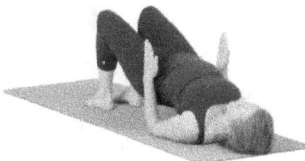

BRIDGE
Shoulders and hips.

***PASSIVE SPINAL TWIST
(both sides)**
Knees and shoulders.

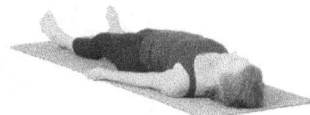

SAVASANA
Rest.

Symmetry Practice: Awaken the Midline

🕐 30 minutes

The goal of this practice is balancing vata by awakening and strengthening the midline in asana. The midline divides our body into its left and right sides and it is through the midline that the 2 sides of our body communicate. Cultivating a clear sense of the midline aligns the body, stabilizes the mind and supports integrated use of the two sides of the body.

Enter this practice by coming into Mountain pose. Use your finger like a pencil to delicately draw a line along the front of your body that traces the midline of your body. Start this line at the point between your eyes, moving along the length of the nose and the continuing along the length of your breastbone, through your navel and down to your pubic bone. Be aware of the spine as running parallel to that line. In each of the following poses cultivate awareness of the midline.

All of the poses in this practice are symmetrical so you can more easily sustain your attention on the midline. As you focus on the midline, alternate between using the entire length of the midline or a small part of it depending on what helps you the most in each pose.

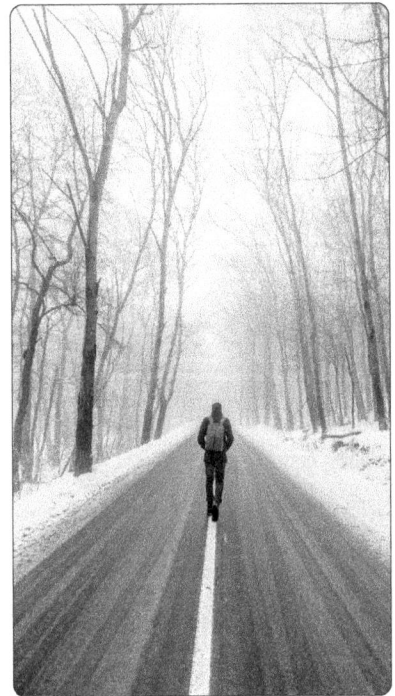

VALENTIN SALJA | UNSPLASH

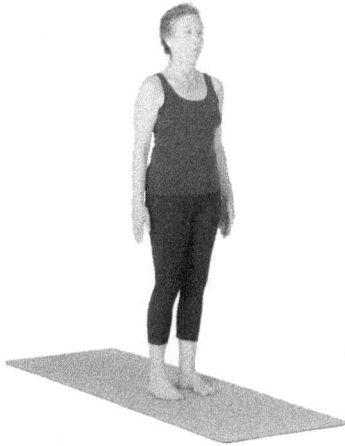

MOUNTAIN

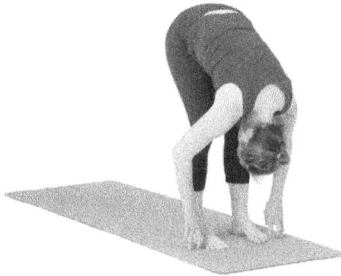

STANDING FORWARD BEND

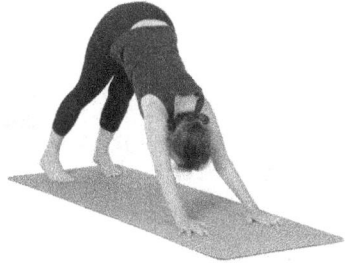

DOWNWARD DOG

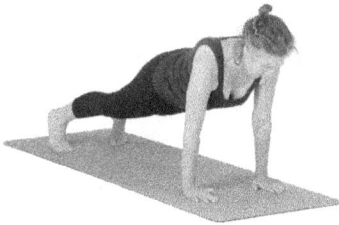

PLANK

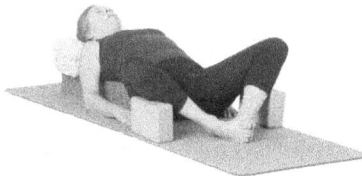

BOUND ANGLE

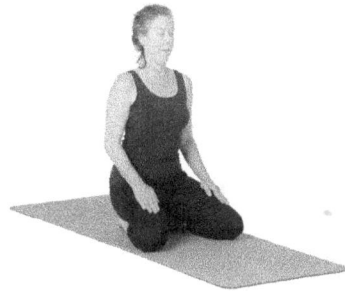

SEATED HERO

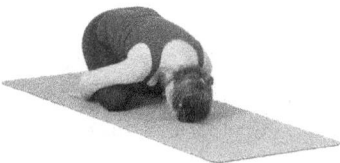

CHILD'S POSE

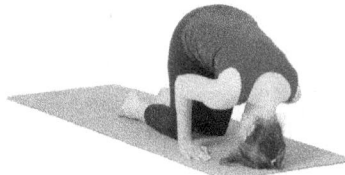

RABBIT

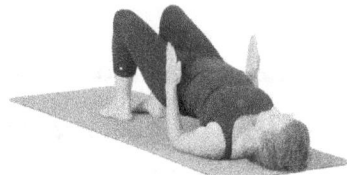

BRIDGE

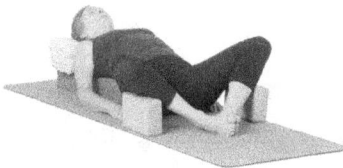

SUPPORTED BOUND ANGLE

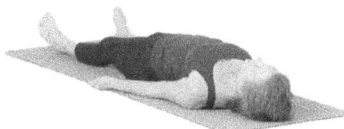

SAVASANA

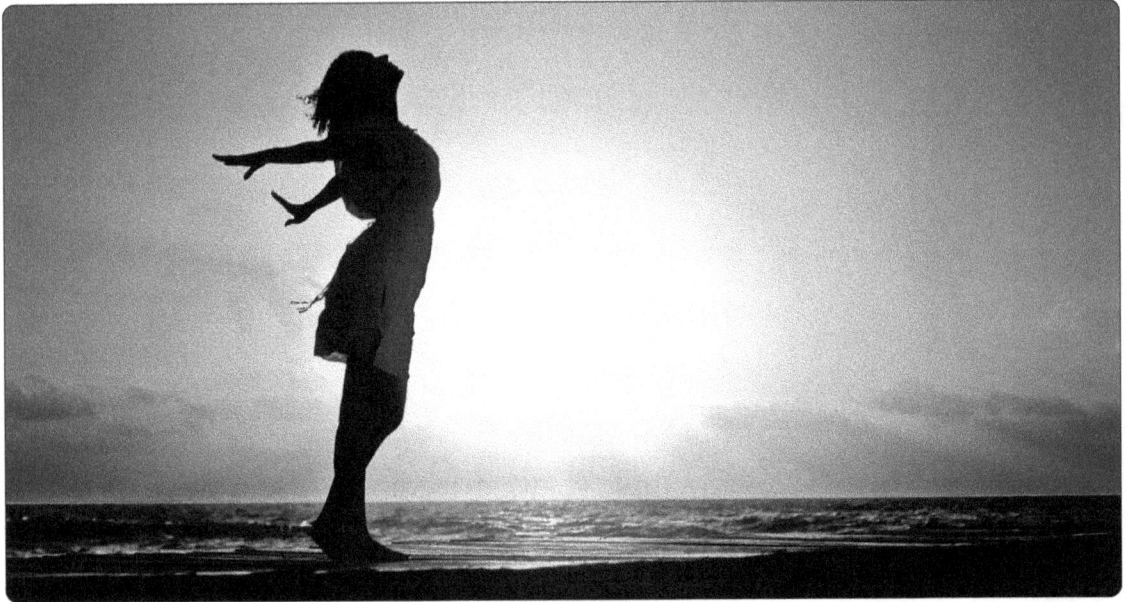

JILL WELLINGTON | PEXELS

Honoring the Sun - A Vedic Prayer

With hands in prayer I face the sun feeling love and joy in my heart.

I reach out and let the sun fill me with warmth.

I bow before the Sun's radiance and place my face to the ground in humble respect.

I lift my face to the sun and remember,

to achieve such heights I must be as the dust of the Earth.

I stretch up towards its light trying to reach the greatest heights, and again surrender.

I stand tall as I remember the true Sun is within me.

"Sūrya is a name for the sun and literally means the sun. In the sun salutation, we bow to the light of the sun. However, the 'light' we are bowing to is the Divine Presence."

— Russill Paul

Sun Salutation

🕐 4 - 6 repetitions

The following Sun Salutation becomes vata balancing when it is done at an easy pace with a focus on the body and breath moving together.

Cultivate a relaxed flow in the sequence with comfortable and satisfying hold in each posture.

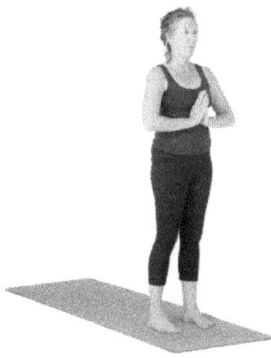

MOUNTAIN
With namaste hands.

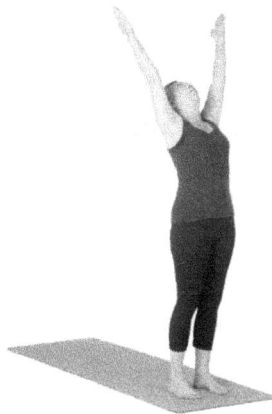

STANDING BACKBEND

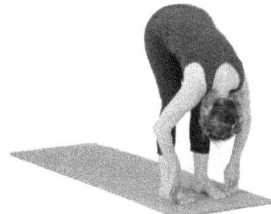

STANDING FORWARD BEND

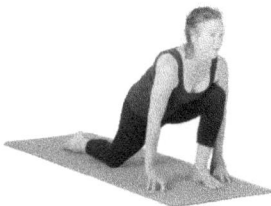

LUNGE

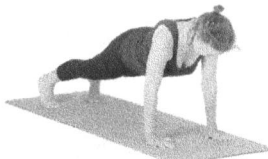

PLANK

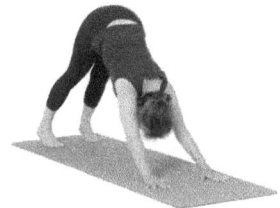

DOWNWARD FACING DOG

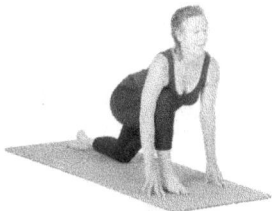

LUNGE

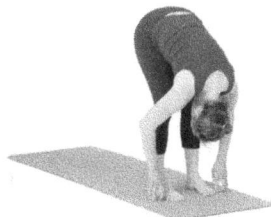

**STANDING
FORWARD BEND**

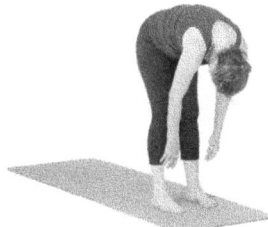

ROLL UP ...

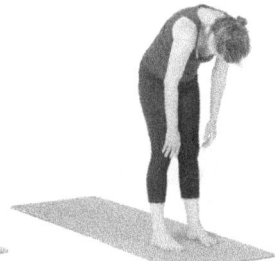

...

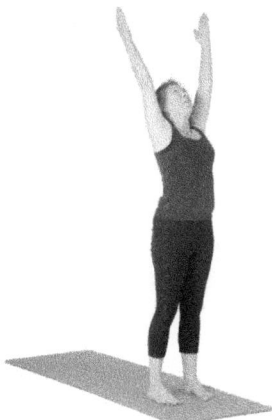

... to STANDING BACKBEND

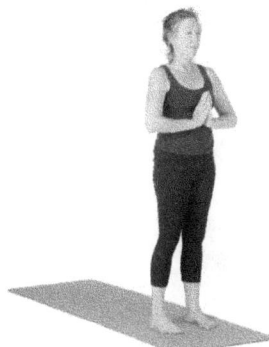

MOUNTAIN
With namaste hands.

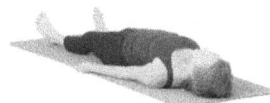

SAVASANA

Prana Practice:
Engage Apana & Samana

🕐 20 minutes

Apana, the downward-moving prana, grounds vata's airy nature. **Samana**, the inward-moving prana, has a gathering and centering action that balances vata's tendency toward dispersion.

In each of the following poses use the exhalation to guide the breath/prana in the direction of the pranic flow that you are cultivating. If you find one of the asanas particularly fruitful for awakening apana or samana, spend more time with it.

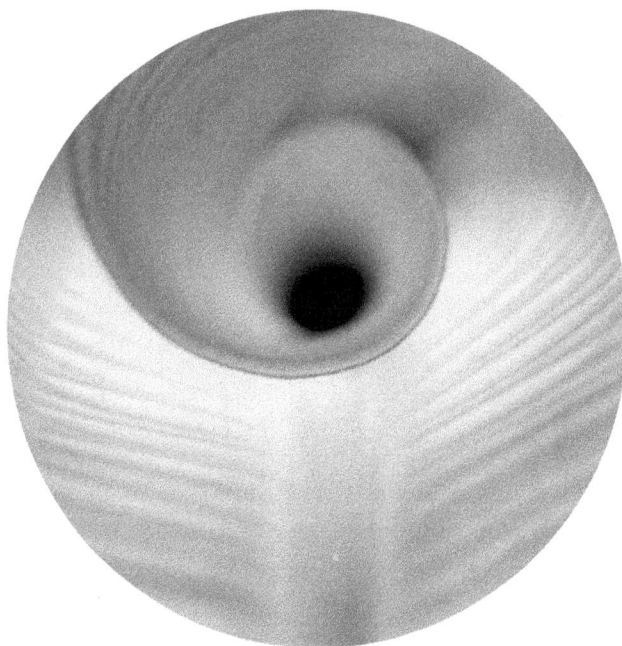

MISUD | DREAMSTIME

Apana (downward-moving prana)   ⏱ 10 minutes

ⓘ **Apana** refresher on page 130.

In each of the following asanas use your exhalation to awaken a downward flow of breath/prana from the top of the pelvis, down through the legs and feet, and into the ground.

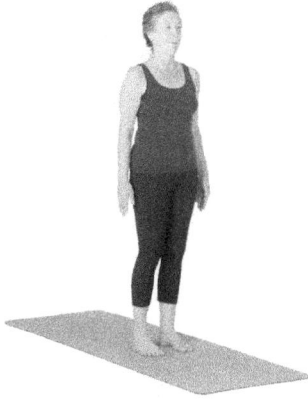

MOUNTAIN

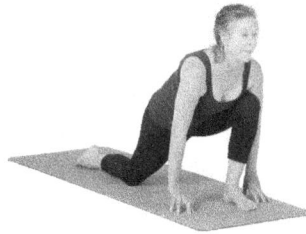

LUNGE
Either straight or bent back knee.

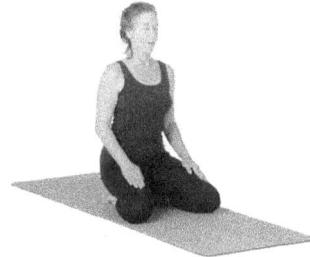

SEATED HERO

Rest in a seated position or Savasana for a few moments before continuing.

—— ✺ ——

Samana (inward-moving prana)   ⏱ 10 minutes

ⓘ **Samana** refresher on page 136.

Focus your attention at the navel and use the exhalation to awaken an inward–drawing action of breath/prana.

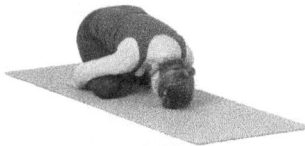

CHILD'S POSE

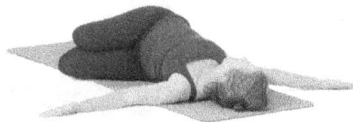

PASSIVE SPINAL TWIST (both sides)

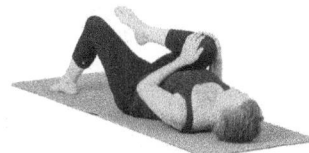

WIND RELIEVING POSE (both sides)

Rest in Savasana to end the practice.

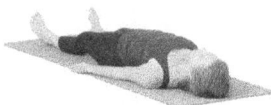

SAVASANA

Breath Practice: Connect to Earth

🕐 5 - 10 minutes

This practice is deeply soothing to the belly and grounding for the whole body.

- ∞ Lie on your stomach with your forehead resting on the backs of your hands. Use a support under your head, chest or belly as needed to make yourself comfortable.

- ∞ Become aware of your breathing and use your exhalations to help your body to release fully into the floor.

- ∞ Bring your attention to your navel. Imagine an umbilical cord growing from your navel and into the earth. The cord can go to any depth that feels comfortable for you.

- ∞ Breathe through this cord. Inhale as if the breath comes from the earth directly into your belly, exhale into the earth.

- ∞ On the exhalation let go into the earth, receiving its support. On the inhalation take in nourishment from the earth, allowing yourself to feel safe and protected.

- ∞ Turn your head to one side and rest, or roll onto your back and rest in Savasana.

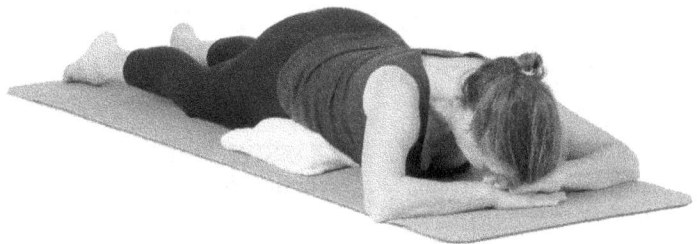

Meditation: 1st Chakra & "Lam"

🕐 5 - 10 minutes

The 1st chakra and its seed mantra *lam* are related to the earth element and so are useful focuses for grounding vata's airy nature. Doing this practice as a meditation for 2 or 3 minutes before or after an asana practice has a lovely vata-balancing effect. Done for 15 - 20 minutes, it is rejuvenating. You can use this practice with mental repetitions as a vata-balancing touchstone during a busy day.

ℹ️ The "a" in all seed mantras is pronounced like the word "some."

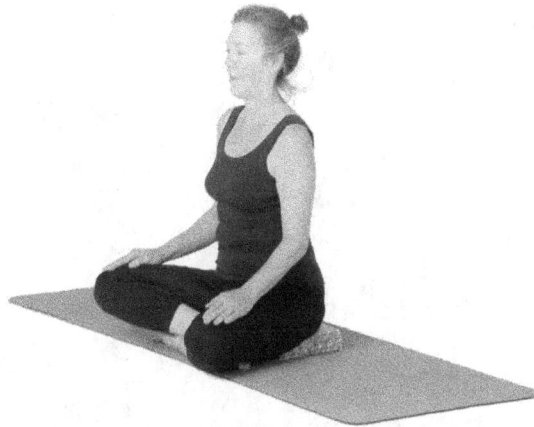

🌀 Find a comfortable seated position and take a few minutes to settle.

🌀 Bring your attention to the area of your tailbone, breathing as if the breath flows in and out through this area.

🌀 Maintain connection to the breath in the tailbone as you vocally or sub-vocally chant *lam*. Place the vibration of the sound in the tailbone.

🌀 If you are doing this as a longer practice, you can alternate between vocalizing and sub-vocalizing *lam* along with periods of rest. The alternating creates a richer experience.

🌀 Sit quietly for a few moments before continuing with your day.

Pitta-Balancing Practices – Keeping Heat in Check

Part of growing up in northern Canada was camping vacations in the mountains and memories of cool evenings by a campfire. My experience of finding the right proximity to a campfire is reminiscent of the sensitivity needed to tend to our internal fire. Feeling chilled I would move closer to the fire only to feel the sharpness of its heat as too hot for me. Moving back from the fire I could easily feel chilled. I was always looking for the right amount of heat.

Tending our internal fire is important for people of all doshic types. Pittas, with their dominance of fire, need to know how to keep their fire from burning too hot. They need to have tools for cooling themselves mentally, physically and emotionally. Developing sensitivity to early signs of fire increase and knowing how to bring themselves back into balance is key to preventing problems that arise from the high heat of disturbed pitta.

Excess vata is often the driving force behind increased pitta. Excess vata acts like a wind fanning the pitta's fire and making it burn hotter. For this reason, becoming familiar with vata-balancing Seeds and Sequences is important for pittas in learning how to keep themselves cool.

In this chapter we offer a variety of pitta-balancing practices. These practices are organized under Pitta-Balancing Practice Seeds and Pitta-Balancing Practice Sequences. The Seeds are pitta-balancing points that can be integrated in your regular practice. The Sequences are structured pitta-balancing yoga practices to learn.

"You have to learn how to listen to your body, going with it and not against it, avoiding all effort or strain."

— *Vanda Scaravelli*

Practice Seeds for Balancing Pitta

Sprinkle one or more of the pitta-balancing Seeds into your asana practice to boost its pitta-balancing effect. For a stronger pitta-balancing effect simply use more Seeds. Maintaining pitta's internal fire burning at an optimal temperature is the goal in balancing pitta.

PHYSICAL SEEDS for BALANCING PITTA

Doshic Home Site refresher on page 105.

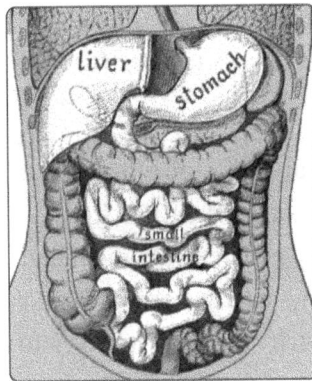

Attend to Pitta Home Site

The stomach, liver and small intestine are the home site of pitta. Reducing tension and maintaining alignment in these organs goes a good distance in keeping pitta balanced.

Cultivate softness in the upper belly just under the diaphragm and in the center of the lower abdomen.

Use gentle twists to give a soothing massage to the stomach, liver and small intestine. If the twist is too strong it will disturb rather than balance pitta.

Gentle, small, supported backbends coupled with easy, relaxed breathing through the pitta organs. If the backbends are too intense they will disturb rather than balance pitta.

PITTA SEEDS

Stay Cool

Cooling is an essential theme for people with a pitta constitution or a pitta disturbance.

Rest for 3-5 minutes in Savasana at the end of a asana practice, particularly if it is a physically demanding practice.	Make restorative asana a regular part of your practice.	When cultivating strength stop short your limit. Pushing to the limit disturbs pitta.

— ✳ —

Connect the Heart to the Arms

All doshas benefit from opening the chest and connecting the arms to the heart. This is especially true for pitta. Softening the chest and heart and allowing heart energy to flow through the arms is an important contribution to pitta balance.

Relax the shoulders and release tension from around the heart.	Allow the warmth of heart energy to flow through the arms, hands and fingers.	Soften the outside of the ribcage on the inhalation and soften the inside of the ribcage on the exhalation.

— ✳ —

Widen & Soften the Lower Back

Pitta's driven personality frequently expresses in them as an overuse of the lumbar spine. Widening and softening the lower back and allowing it to be receptive to the breath releases the tension from an overused lumbar spine. This is beneficial in both yoga and daily life.

Let the sacrum give into gravity and drop toward the ground.	Allow the muscles of the lower back to relax away from the spine.	Support the widening of the lower back by encouraging the front lower ribs to move toward each other and move slightly in the direction of the pelvis.

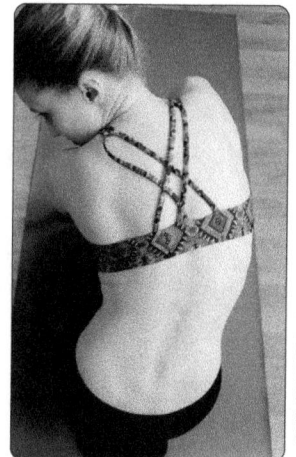

GMB FITNESS | UNSPLASH

Reduce Effort

Pitta's bias toward enjoying strong-focused activity makes them prone to using more effort than is needed for the activity at hand. Learning to reduce effort helps to keep their pitta balanced and makes their actions more efficient.

Work at less than maximum capacity in asana.	Reduce effort by a particular percentage. Start by reducing effort by 10% and working up to 50%.	Look to and release tension from different areas of the body during asana, for example legs, arms and breath.

---❂---

Quiet the Eyes

The eyes have a concentration of fire energy. This makes the eyes a good focus for a pitta-reducing practice.

Relax the muscles around the eyes, and let the eyes release into the backs of the sockets.	Let the eyes descend in the direction of the heart.	Soften the eyes and awaken peripheral vision.

"Yoga is the golden key that unlocks the door to peace, tranquility, and joy."

— B. K. S. Iyengar

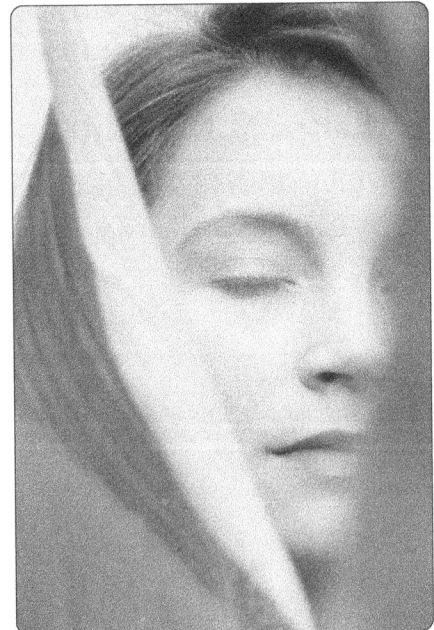

ALINA VILCHENKO | PEXELS

PITTA SEEDS

BREATH/ENERGETIC SEEDS
for BALANCING PITTA

Breath

Cultivating cooling and soothing qualities in the breath is important for pittas. Cooling pranayamas such as Sitali and Sitkari* are also great for pitta balancing and can be used together with the following pitta-balancing breath practices.

Cultivate long easy exhalations and passive inhalations.	Breathe as if the breath is entering and leaving the body through the pores of the skin.	Integrate Sitali and Sitkari* pranayama into asana, or do at the end of your practice.

see Appendix, page 229

Prana

Apana, the downward-moving prana, is essential energetic support for healthy pitta. So too is a balanced interplay between inward-moving **samana** and outward-moving **vyana**.

Apana refresher on page 130.

Samana refresher on page 136.

Vyana refresher on page 134.

Cultivate the flow of apana by using the exhalation to awaken a downward breath-flow from the pelvis, through the legs and feet, and into the ground.	Cultivate a sensitive balance between samana and vyana. Connect the inhalation to vyana as an outward flow from the heart and connect the exhalation to the inward draw of samana at the navel.	Soften the skin away from the muscles to allow ease in the outward movement of vyana and the inward movement of samana.

Elements

Water and earth are the elemental energies to engage for balancing pitta.

Awaken a gentle whole-body fluidity using an easy paced, simple version of Sun Salutation.	Cultivate sensitive aware-ness of the contact of your feet on the floor as if burrowing your feet into soft, cool sand.	Maintain soft attention on breathing as if the breath is moving in and out of the body through the pelvis (1st and 2nd chakras).

MENTAL/EMOTIONAL SEEDS
for BALANCING PITTA

Intention

When disturbed, pitta's fiery nature expresses in being irritable, sharp-tongued and competitive. Cultivating compassion, contentment and surrender are important aspects of pitta balancing. You can use these as Seeds during an asana practice to increase its pitta-balancing effect.

Release irritability on the exhalation and receive compassion on the inhalation.	Focus on contentment as the goal of an asana practice.	Practice surrendering your body into the asanas, and meet any physical or emotional resistance with acceptance and kindness.

— ❖ —

Imagery

Pittas tend to be visual people so imagery can work well for them in asana, pranayama and meditation. Cooling is the primary need for pitta people so cooling images are a good resource for pitta balancing.

Imagine/sense doing your practice in a gentle, cooling waterfall. Allow the cooling of the water to permeate your body.	Imagine/sense doing your practice in a pleasantly cool evening under a silvery moon. Take the coolness of the image into your experience of the asana.	As you exhale release heat from your body, as you inhale imagine the temperature of your body drops down a degree.

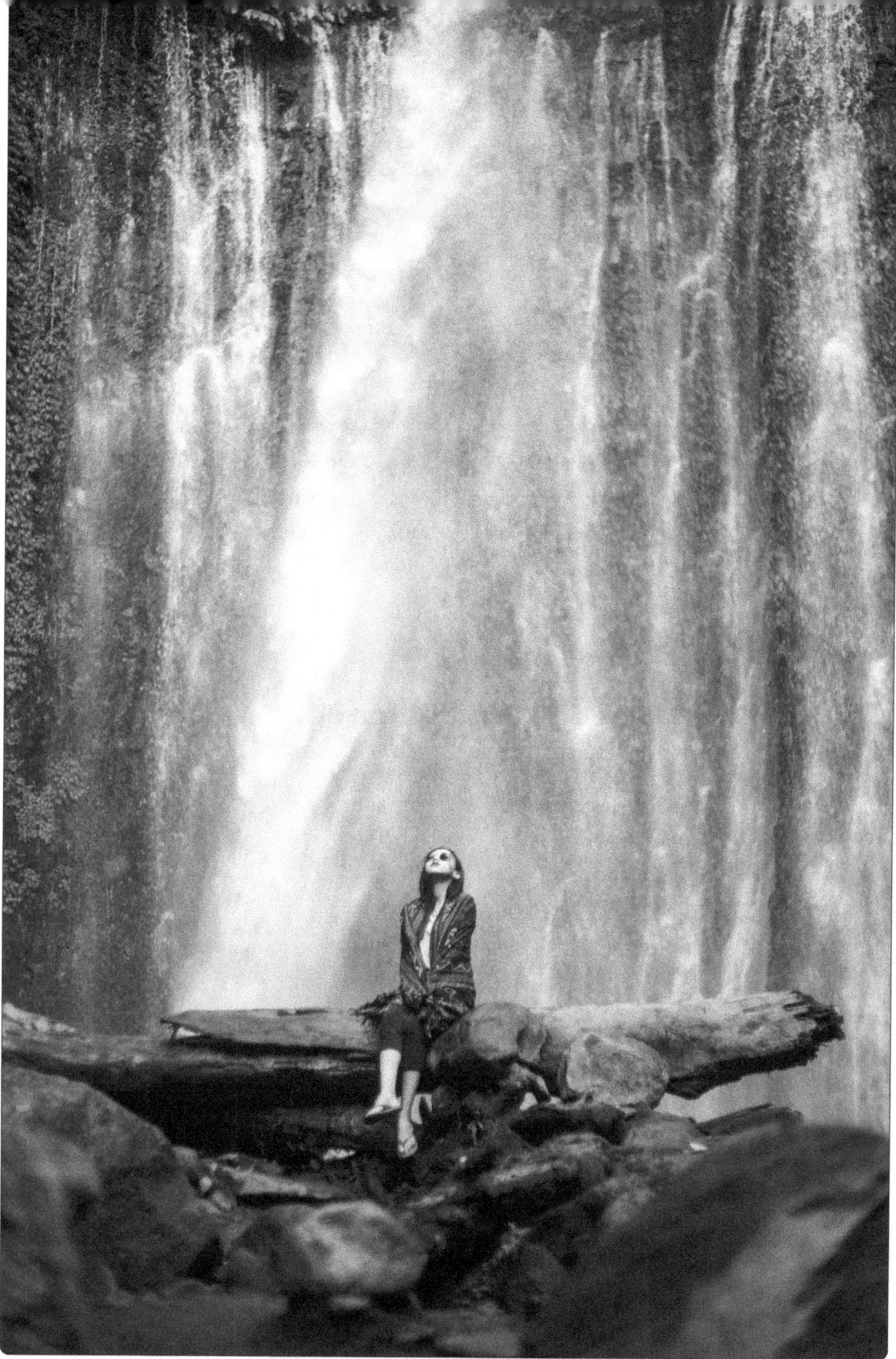

Practice Sequences for Balancing Pitta

Home Site Practice for Pitta

🕐 25 minutes

Balancing pitta using its home site focuses on releasing tension in the diaphragm, relaxing the muscles of both the upper abdomen and center of the lower abdomen, and very gently massaging the pitta organs.

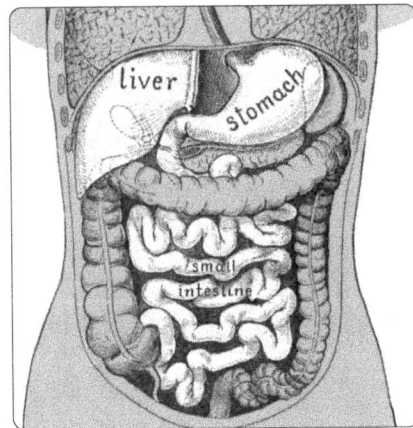

Use the image of the pitta organs to refresh your memory about the location and shape of the stomach, liver and small intestine. In doing the following practice, focus on the stomach, liver and small intestine; or on the upper abdomen from the bottom of the breastbone to the navel and the center of the lower abdomen. Both ways of focusing are equally effective.

Each asana has a suggestion for using your awareness to enhance the action of the pose. Keep in mind that reducing effort is an essential component of a pitta-reducing practice.

PITTA SEQUENCES

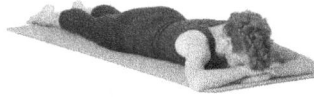

CROCODILE
Sense the movement of your breathing and use each exhalation to soften the upper abdomen.

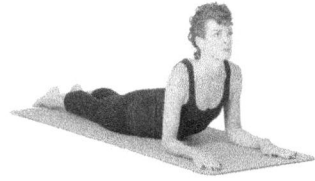

BABY or SPHINX COBRA
Lift head and chest just high enough to feel a gentle opening of the pitta organs. Sense the movement of your breathing massaging the organs and the muscles around them.

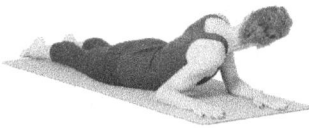

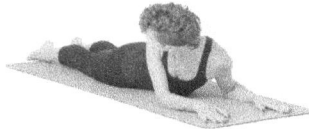

BABY COBRA or SPHINX COBRA with TWIST (both sides)
Come back into Cobra, hold for a few moments to settle into the pose. Initiating from the upper abdomen (pitta area), rotate your spine, torso and neck as you look toward your feet. Hold for a minute, breathing into the pitta organs then come back to Cobra. Hold Cobra for a few moments then repeat on the other side.

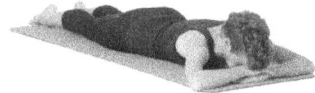

CROCODILE
Let the breath gently massage the pitta organs, the spine behind the organs and muscles around them.

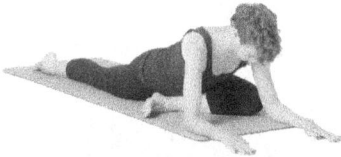

BABY PIGEON (both sides)
The front leg pitta organs are being lightly compressed while the back-leg pitta organs are being lightly stretched. Breathe softly into either or both sides of the pitta organs.

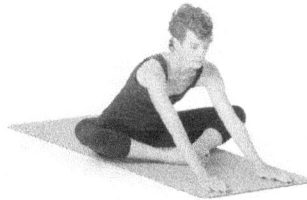

BOUND ANGLE with slight FORWARD BEND
Breathe into the entire pitta organ area — organs, lower ribs and lower back spine.

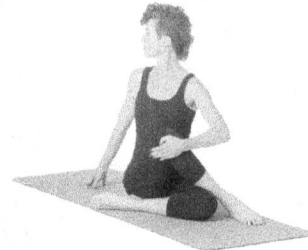

SEATED TWIST
Sense/image the organs spiraling softly. Encourage this softening with gentle breathing into the organs.

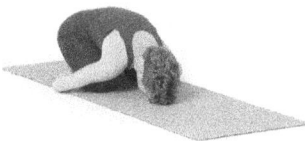

CHILD'S POSE
Breathe in the back at the level of the stomach, liver and small intestine.

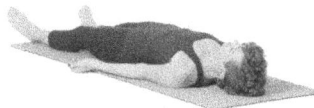

SAVASANA

Release Lower Back Practice

🕐 20 minutes

Releasing lower back tension and mobilizing the back lower ribs eases the muscular overwork that is usually present in pittas in this area of the body. The goal of this practice is threefold:

- initiate breath in the lower back
- widen the lower back by releasing the muscles away from the spine
- cultivate an easy, peaceful breath that flows through the lower back, lumbar spine and lower back ribs.

Each asana has an additional suggestion to enhance this goal.

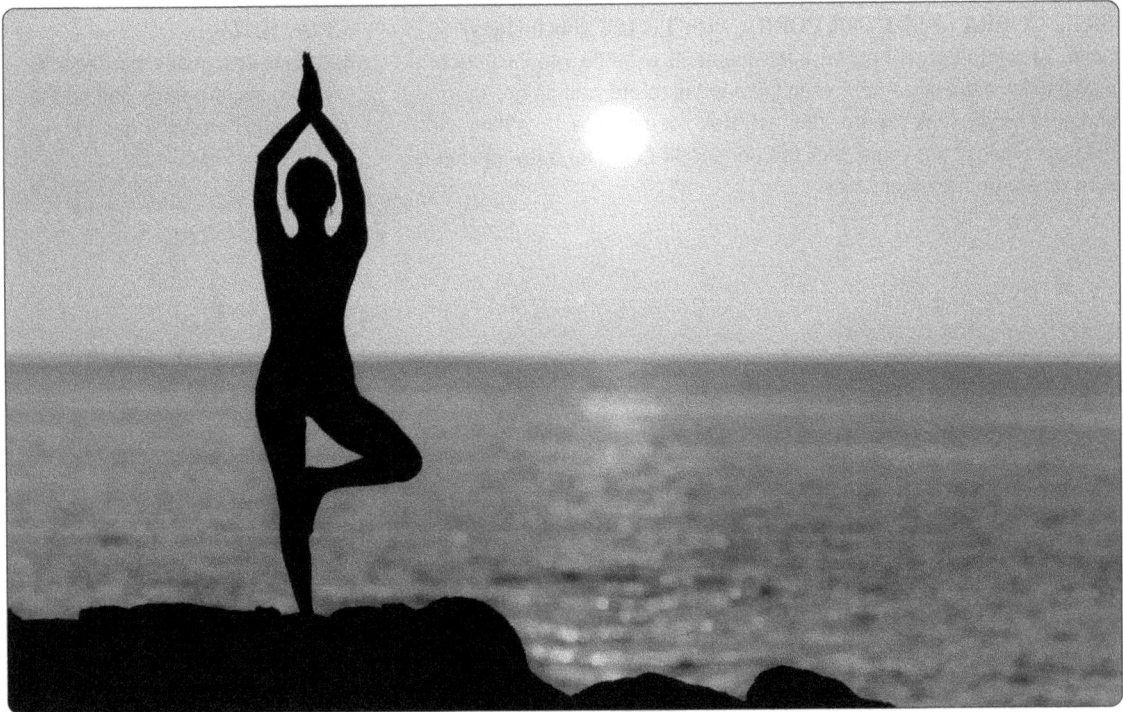

CEDRIC LIM AH TOCK | PEXELS

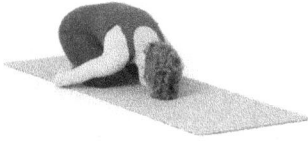

CHILD'S POSE
Sense the movement of breath in your lower back.

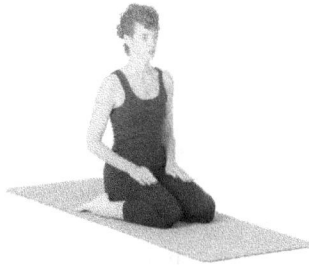

SEATED HERO Inhale. Let the lower back widen by releasing the lower back muscles away from the spine; exhale while lightly maintaining the lower back width.

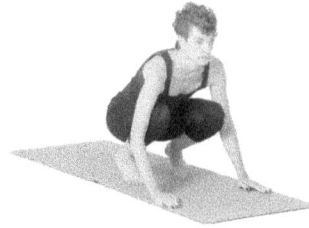

SQUAT
Breathe into and soften the area where the lower back meets the thoracic spine.

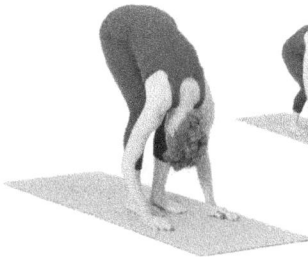

FORWARD BEND
Allow the lower back spine to release.

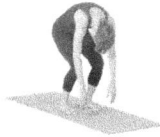

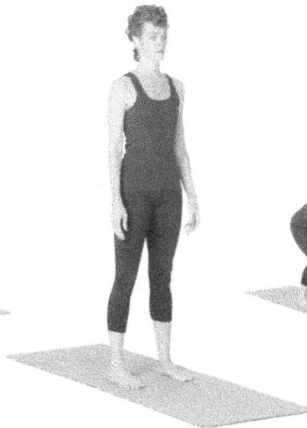

MOUNTAIN
With attention on rounding the lower back spine, roll up to standing. Reverse these movements and exhale as you return to Squat.

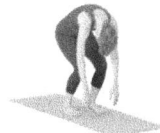

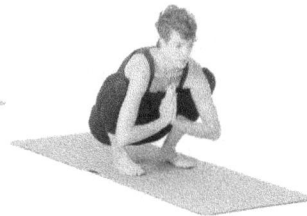

SQUAT
Breathe into and soften the muscles of the lower back.

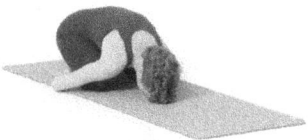

CHILD'S POSE
Fold forward into Child's Pose, focusing on breath moving through and widening the lower back.

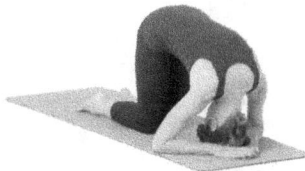

RABBIT
Relax, round and lengthen the whole the spine.

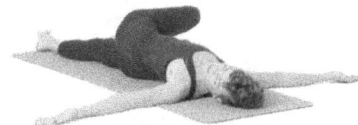

PASSIVE SPINAL TWIST (both sides) Use the breath to soften the lower back on the side that is closest to the floor.

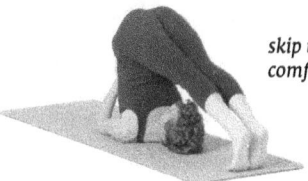

skip unless easy and comfortable

PLOUGH POSE
Soften the entire spine and focus the breath in the lower back and bottom ribs.

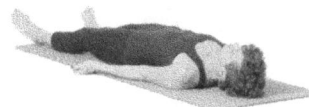

SAVASANA

Joints Practice: A Still Point in the Joints

🕐 25 minutes

This practice cultivates a soft, expansive awareness to counteract pitta's tendency to use a narrow, hard focus. In each of the following poses cultivate a tiny point of stillness in the center of the joints.

Allow all the points of stillness to come into your awareness simultaneously as you would when viewing a constellation of stars in the night sky. The points come into your awareness, rather than your awareness going outward toward the points. The softer and more receptive is your awareness, the more easily you will be able to receive the points.

Each of the poses has suggested joints on which to focus. Feel free to use fewer joints. As this process becomes more familiar you can include as many joints as you like. The joints in parentheses can be deleted if you prefer to work with two joints.

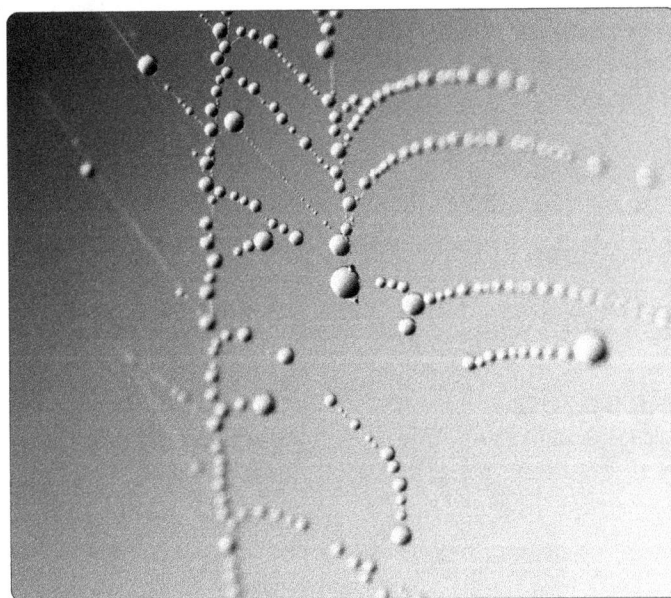

ROBIN MELLIGER | UNSPLASH

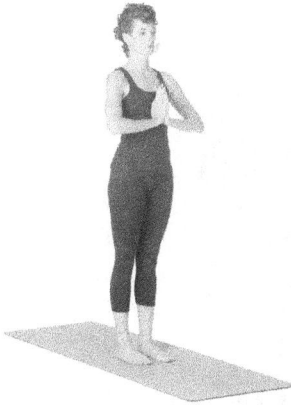

MOUNTAIN with NAMASTE HANDS
Ankles and wrists.

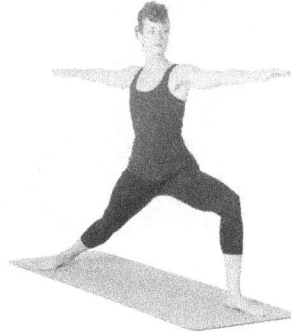

HERO II (both sides)
Hips and shoulders.

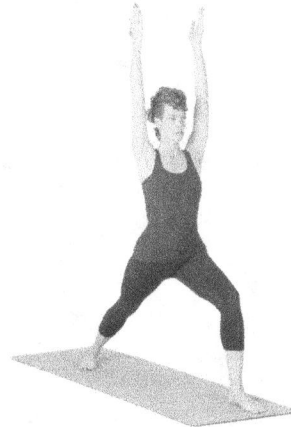

HERO I (both sides)
Shoulders, (elbows) and wrists.

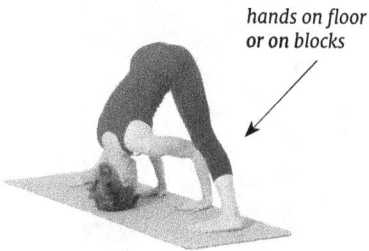

hands on floor or on blocks

STANDING WIDE-ANGLE FORWARD BEND
Hips and ankles.

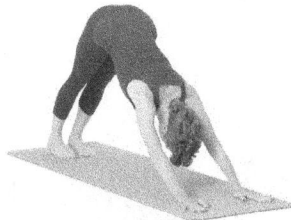

DOWNWARD FACING DOG
Hips, shoulders and (ankles).

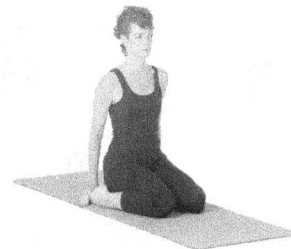

SEATED HERO
Ankles, knees and (hips).

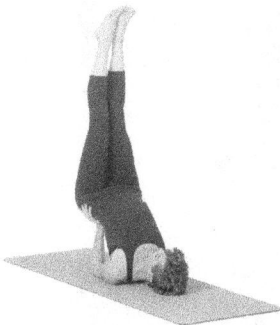

HALF SHOULDER STAND
Shoulders, wrists and (ankles).

skip unless easy and comfortable

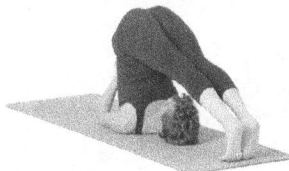

PLOUGH
Shoulder, hips and (ankles).

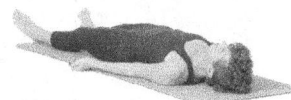

SAVASANA

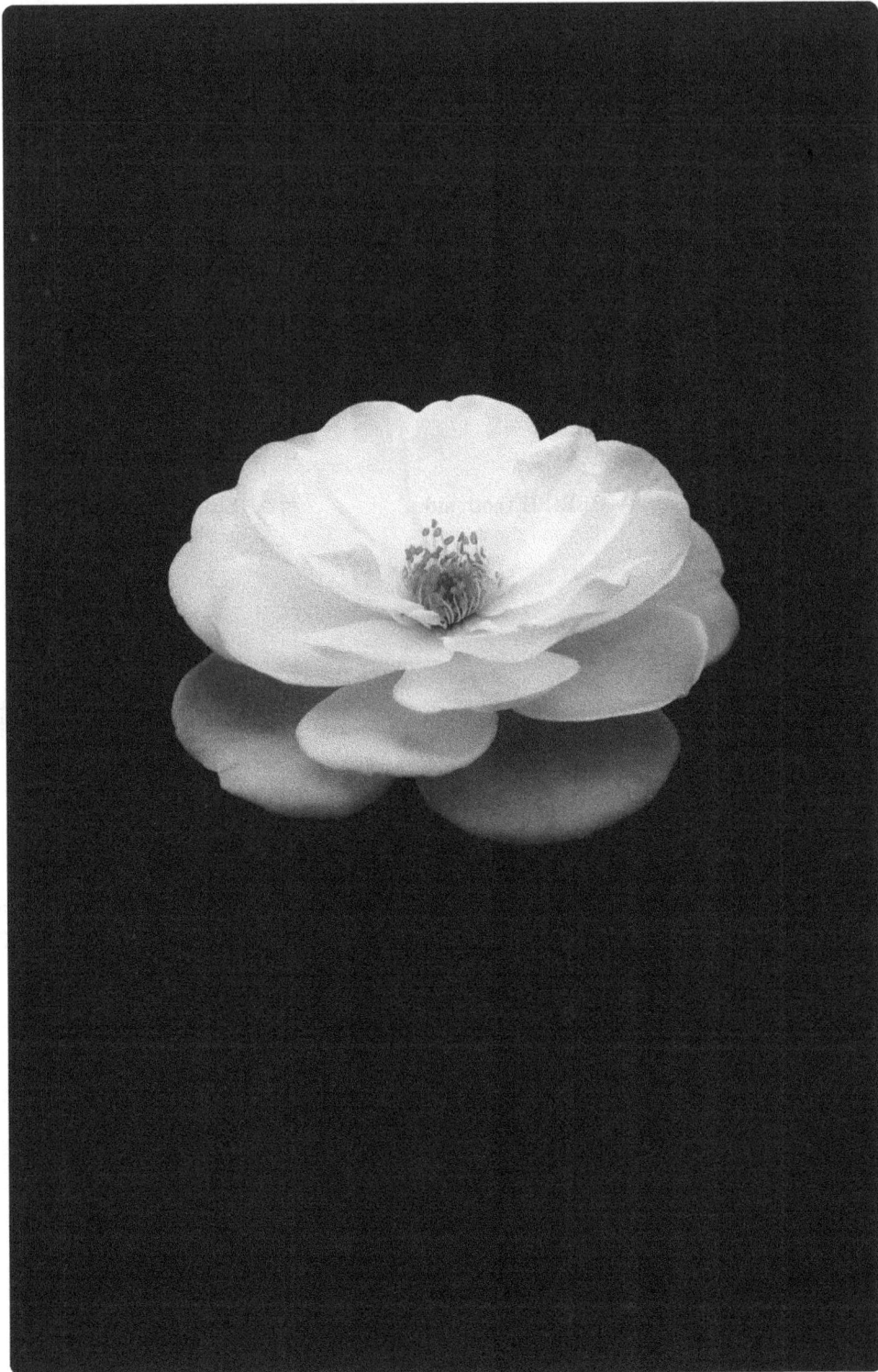

Forward Bends: A Cooling Practice

🕐 20 minutes

Forward Bends are the bread-and-butter of cooling practices. The following is a simple and effective practice.

In each pose yield slowly and deeply into the folding of the hip joints. Release tension along the spine and relax the muscles of the back away from the spine.

Relax the eyes deeply, letting them move toward the backs of the sockets, and downward in the direction of the heart.

These poses can be done with or without supports.

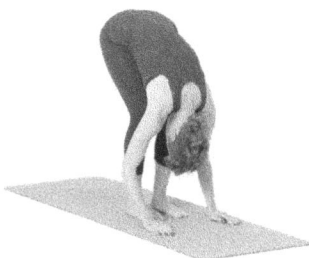

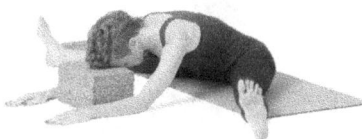

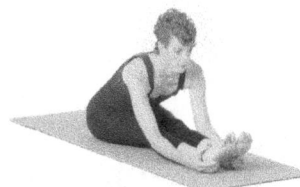

STANDING FORWARD BEND

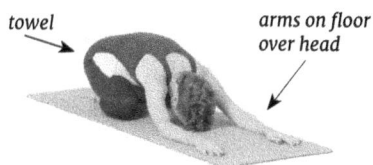

towel
arms on floor over head

SUPPORTED CHILD'S POSE

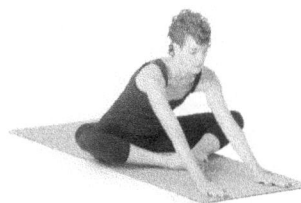

BOUND ANGLE FORWARD BEND

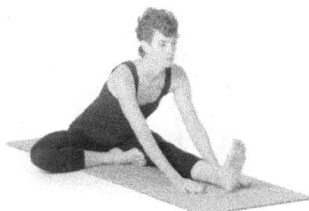

HEAD TO KNEE (both sides)
With or without support.

WIDE ANGLE FORWARD BEND
With or without support.

STRETCH-of-the-BACK-BODY FORWARD BEND

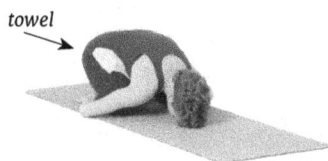

towel

SUPPORTED CHILD'S POSE
Arms alongside the legs.

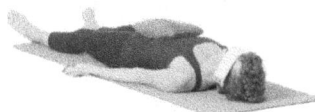

SAVASANA with EYE BAG and SAND BAG

Prana Practice:
Engage Apana & Vyana/Samana

The downward-moving energy of apana grounds pitta helping to keep pitta's fire from burning too hot or spreading too far. Balancing vyana and samana softens the sharpness and intensity to which pittas are prone.

This is a two-part practice with the first part focusing on apana and the second part on vyana and samana

Apana refresher on page **130**.

Apana (downward-moving prana)

🕐 10 minutes

In the following asanas, as you exhale sense/imagine your breath flowing downward through the pelvis, legs, feet, and into the earth. Let the inhalation come in on its own.

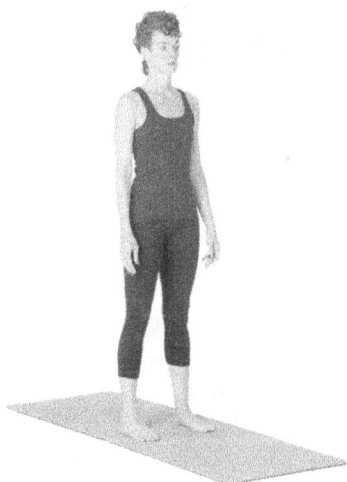

MOUNTAIN POSE & HERO I or II
In these standing poses pay particular attention to cultivating the downward flow through the hip joints, knees and ankles.

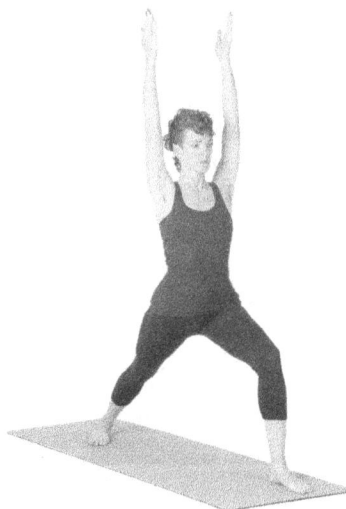

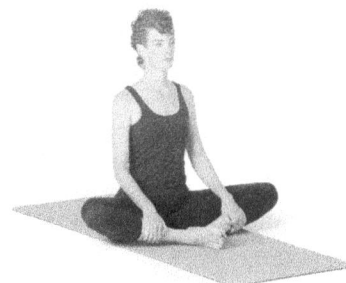

BOUND ANGLE
Sense/image apana moving into the earth through the sitz bones.

Rest briefly before continuing. If your time is constrained you can stop here and do vyana and samana at a later time.

PITTA SEQUENCES

Vyana and Samana
(outward- and inward-moving prana)
⏱ 10 minutes

The first of the following three poses focuses on awakening samana, the second on awakening vyana and the third on awakening them in relation to each other.

ℹ
Samana refresher on page 136.

Vyana refresher on page 134.

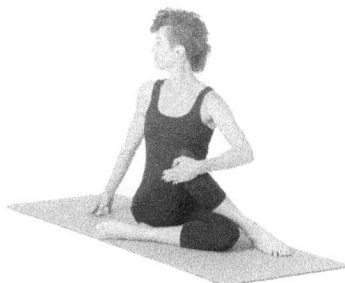

SEATED SPINAL TWIST (both sides)
Evoking samana, bring your attention to the navel and on the exhalation create an inward-spiraling action from the navel toward the spine.

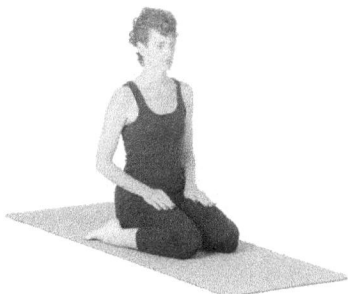

SEATED HERO
Evoking vyana, bring your attention to your heart. Exhale as if the breath moves in an outward-dispersing action from the heart, flowing equally in all directions toward and beyond the surface of the body.

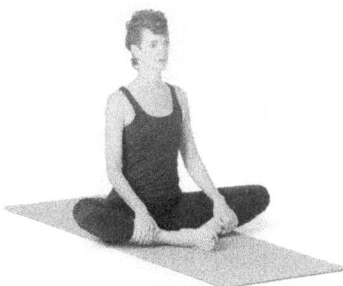

BOUND ANGLE
Evoking samana and vyana, exhale as if the breath flows in an inward-spiraling action from the navel toward the spine. On the inhalation, feel the breath starting in the heart and flowing outward to and beyond the entire surface of the body. Cultivate an easy interplay between these.

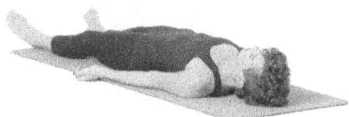

SAVASANA
Rest in Savasana to end the practice.

Breath Practice: A Cooling Breath

🕐 6 - 8 minutes

This practice combines the cooling of Sitkari* pranayama with a focus on the 1st chakra. The first chakra is related to the earth element.

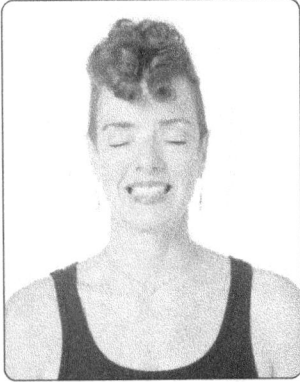

🔥 Sit or lie comfortably giving yourself a minute or so to settle. On each exhalation release your body's weight into the earth.

🔥 Holding your teeth together with lips stretched sideways toward your ears, inhale slowly and softly through all of the spaces between your teeth. Let the inhalation enter like a cooling spray that flows through your whole body as if touching each cell with a cool breeze. As you exhale through the spaces between the teeth, imagine heat flowing out of your body.

🔥 Breathe in this way for 2 minutes.

🔥 Relax for 1 minute with your attention resting on the 1st chakra in the area of the tailbone.

🔥 Repeat Sitkari 2 minutes.

🔥 Relax for a minute resting your attention on the 1st chakra.

see Appendix, page 229

"Breathing in, I calm body and mind.
Breathing out, I smile.
Dwelling in the present moment,
I know this is the only moment. "

— *Thich Nhat Hanh*

Meditation: Cooling Nature Imagery

🕐 7 - 10 minutes

This meditation uses nature imagery for cooling pitta.

🔥 Sit in a comfortable meditation position or supported reclining position.

🔥 Relax your eyes toward the backs of the sockets and downward toward the heart.

🔥 Imagine you are sitting beside a cool, peaceful mountain lake or by a gentle waterfall. It can be a place with which you are familiar or a creation of your imagination. The important thing is that it is a cool spot in nature and that it is a place in which you can feel safe.

🔥 Rest for a minute or more, soaking in the energy of this spot.

🔥 Bring your attention to your breathing.

🔥 As you inhale, take in and deeply absorb that cool, peaceful energy, as if into every cell. As you exhale, let your body/mind yield more and more fully into a sense of ease.

🔥 Rest for a minute or more before continuing with your day.

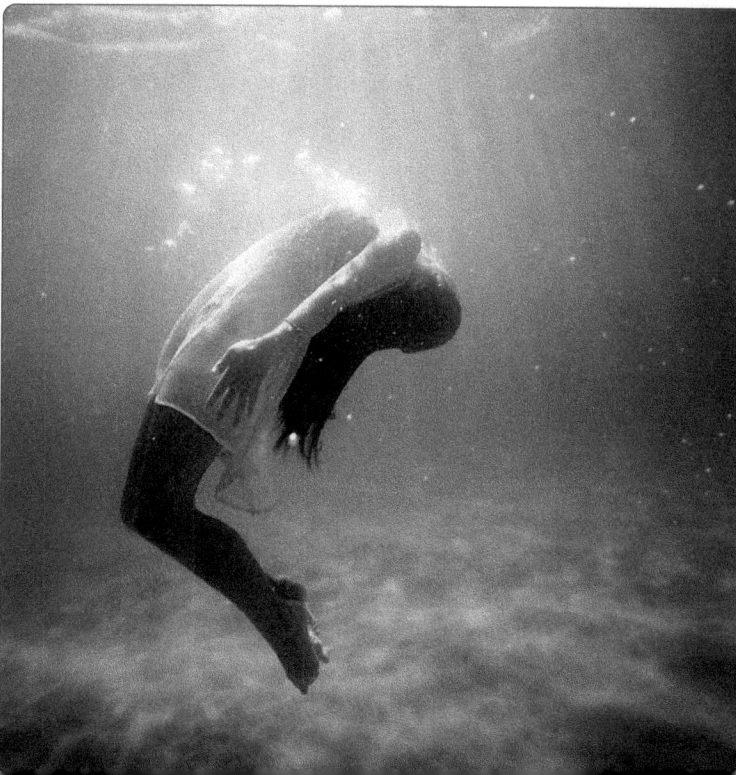

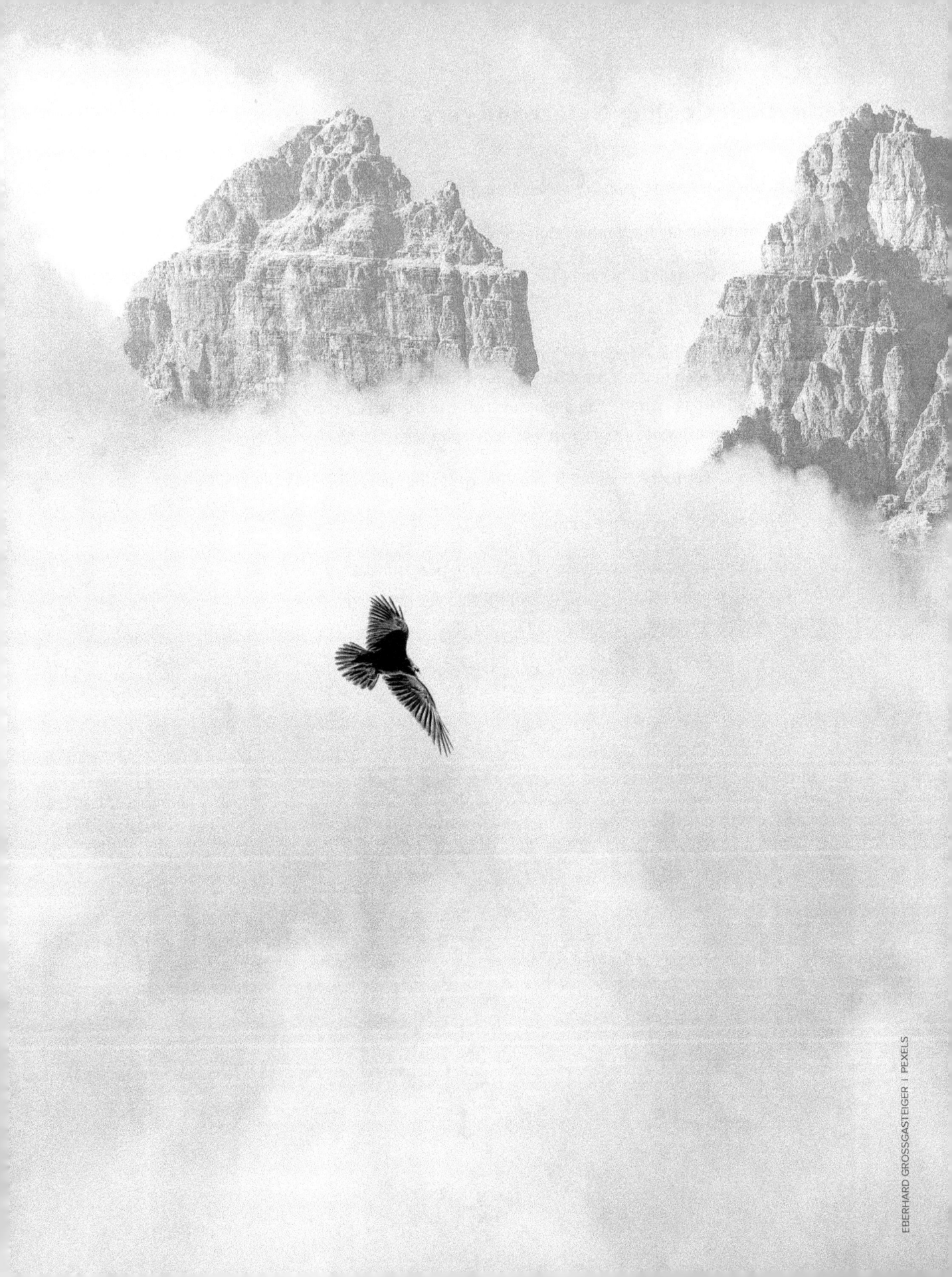

Kapha-Balancing Practices - Mobilizing Earth

I grew up in the city but spent summers on the farm of my relatives. During these summer visits I developed a connection to the earth and an awareness of the different stages of growing crops and gardens. The first step was preparing the earth by tilling it with hoes, rakes, picks, shovels or large machinery. Tilling turned over and loosened the earth so it would support the growth of the seeds that would be planted. As the seeds grew into plants they were stressed so they would become strong. I remember a conversation at the dinner table about the sweetness and tastiness of a vegetable being dependent on the plant being stressed.

As a combination of earth and water, kapha has great potential for fruitfulness. Kaphas are considered the most fortunate of the doshas because they tend naturally to have good health, physical strength and compassion. Like farmland, however, kaphas's earth needs to be tilled; it needs to be turned over and loosened if kaphas are to enjoy the full expression of their natural gifts.

Kaphas need to challenge themselves in order to fully bloom. They need practices that increase their internal heat, mobilize their body and awaken their upward-moving energy. The gravity-bound earth and water nature of kaphas needs to be stressed in order to access its full potential.

In this chapter we offer a variety of kapha-balancing practices. These practices are organized under Kapha-Balancing Practice Seeds and Kapha-Balancing Practice Sequences. The Seeds are kapha-balancing points that can be integrated in your regular practice. The Sequences are structured kapha-balancing yoga practices to learn.

Practice Seeds for Balancing Kapha

Sprinkle one or more of the following kapha-balancing Seeds through your asana practice to boost its kapha-balancing effect. For a stronger effect simply use more Seeds.

PHYSICAL SEEDS for BALANCING KAPHA

Attend to Kapha Home Site

Doshic Home Site refresher on page 113.

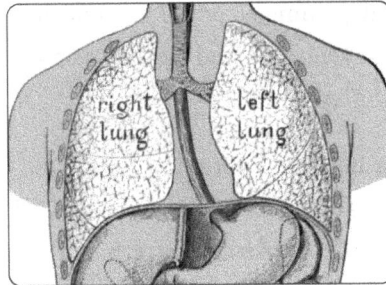

The lungs are the home site of kapha. Kaphas have a propensity for slow digestion and lung congestion so a little extra attention on a regular basis given to stimulating the lungs is good preventive support for keeping kaphas healthy.

Cultivate backbends emphasizing the stretch through the ribcage, chest and lungs.

Use deep twists to massage the stomach and the bottom of the lungs.

Lift and open the ribcage and powerfully reach the arms in Hero poses.

Generate Heat

Kaphas elementally have no fire thus are cool and weak on transformative energy. Heating practices are a necessary part of keeping kapha healthy.

Do 25 - 35 minutes of Sun Salutation or other vinyasa.	Do a series of backbends that build safely in intensity.	Activate the abdomen with Agni Sara* and Uddiyana Bandha.*

— ✺ —

Create Space

Kaphas' density gives them an enviable strength, but their density also expresses in stubbornness and an inability to change. Space lightens this density and air provides it with mobility, helping them develop permeability and awakening their capacity to change.

Enliven the cavities of the head by lifting the pharynx and awakening the space in the mouth and nasal cavities. Lightening the head in this way lightens the whole body.	Awaken and stretch the fingers, hands, toes and feet; encourage the maximum extension of limbs into space.	Create space in all of the joints of the body, particularly through the ribcage and spine.

— ✺ —

Increase Physical Challenge

Strong physical actions are good antidotes to kapha's heaviness. The strength of challenge that kaphas need is best cultivated in digestible bites so it can become a habit.

Develop long, strong and vital holds.	Make time in your practice for exploring increasingly advanced asanas.	Challenge yourself in gravity with standing poses, balance poses and inversions.

See Appendix, page 230

Stimulate the Senses

The eyes are related to pitta and so eye focuses can be used to raise heat in kapha. The ears are related to space and so hearing can be used to lighten kapha.

Cultivate a steady, sharp focus on different actions or structural alignments of the body.

Start a practice by listening into the space around you as if to hear a subtle sound within it. Maintain this enlivened listening throughout a practice.

Use Lion pose to vitalize the tongue, mouth, lungs and upper stomach.

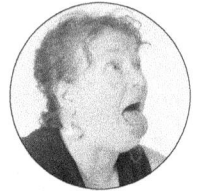

Engage the Joints

Working with joints is a powerful access into influencing the whole body. Gradually expand your capacity to hold more joints in your awareness at the same time. This enlivens the body/mind.

Open space inside the joints.

Stretch through and across the joints, taking care to not lock or hyper-extend them.

In Hero poses, vitalize the whole body by being aware of the center of the joints as points in a constellation that are simultaneously moving away from each other.

TALLIK I DREAMSTIME

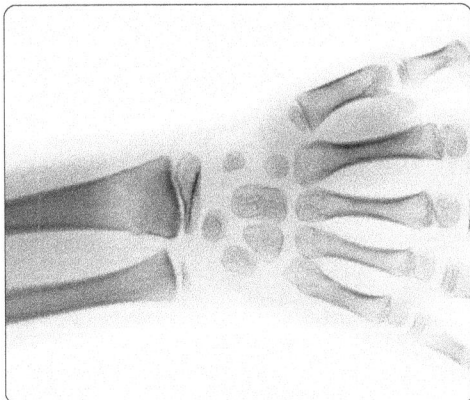

BREATH/ENERGETIC SEEDS
for BALANCING KAPHA

Breath

Kaphas need heating breathwork and pranayama for their heating and stimulating effects.

Focus on increasing inhalations to expand the lungs, increase energy and stimulate the nervous system.	Enjoy daily Kapalabhati and Bastrika.* They can be included during holds in asana.	Maintain awareness of the skin during pranayama inhaling — filling your body to the skin and beyond; exhaling — maintaining a sense of enlivened skin.

Prana

Udana and Vyana/Samana are of particular benefit for kapha balancing.

ℹ️ **Pranas** refresher on page 132.

Exhale, gather and compress the breath into the navel to awaken heat (samana). Inhale, distribute the heat through the whole body and a bit into the space around it.	Use Lion pose to stimulate the mouth and tongue and clarify udana.	Inhale through the heart and exhale through the crown of the head (udana).

Elements

Elemental energies that benefit kapha are fire, air and space.

Cultivate a sharp focus by meditating on the tip of a candle flame.	The continuous movement of vinyasas stimulates the air element.	In Savasana, imagine that the body is completely empty.

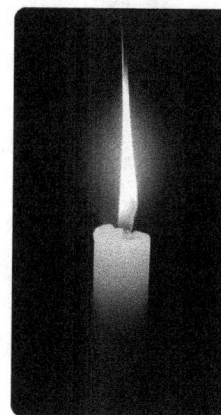

MARC IGNACIO | UNSPLASH

see Appendix, page 228

MENTAL/EMOTIONAL SEEDS
for BALANCING KAPHA

Intention

Kaphas tend to hold on to things — emotions, people and objects. Create a simple and clear intention for letting go of these things. At the beginning of your practice take a quiet moment to repeat this intention to yourself, either out loud or as a thought. Then:

Untie and release grief on the exhalation.	Say goodbye to the past on the exhalation and receive the present on the inhalation.	Open your body, mind and heart to lightness and joy.

---❖---

Imagery

Imagery does not come as easily to kaphas as it does to vatas and pittas. Finding a photo of fire can be used in place of creating a mental image.

Imagine a fire in your solar plexus. Imagine the asanas in your practice as feeding and strengthening that fire.	Inhale into the navel center, let its fire heat the breath, exhale through the space between the eyes.	Invite a mental state that is as light and clear as air at the top of a mountain.

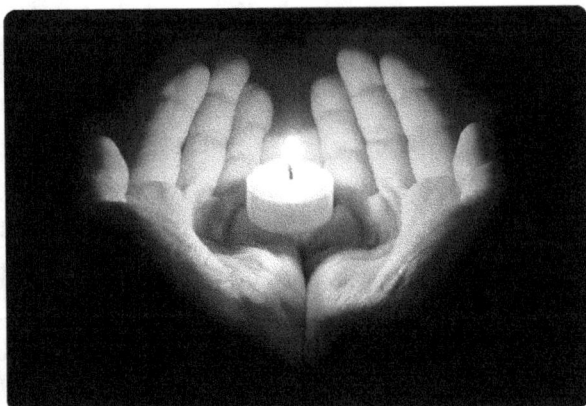

DYOMA | DREAMSTIME

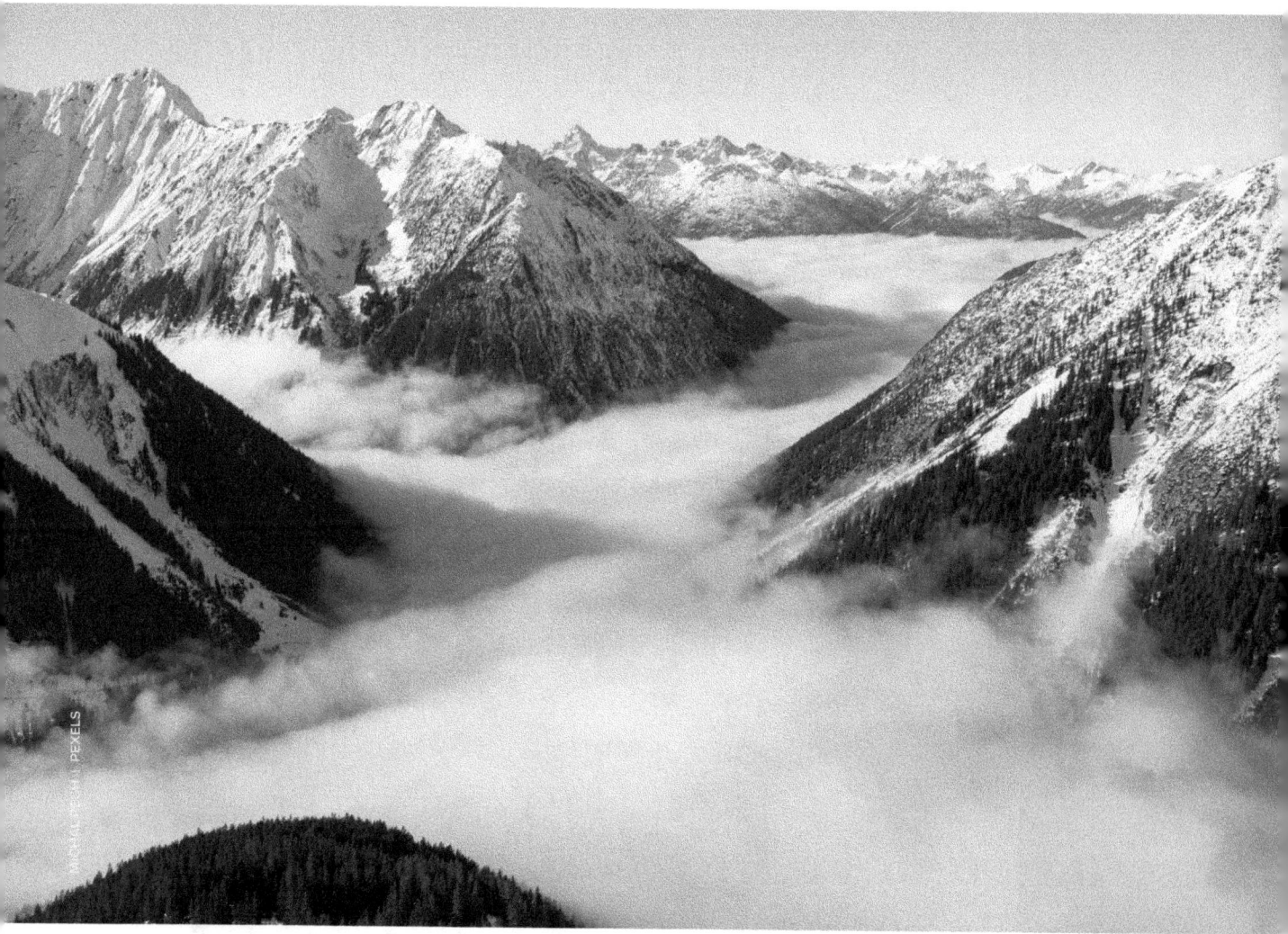

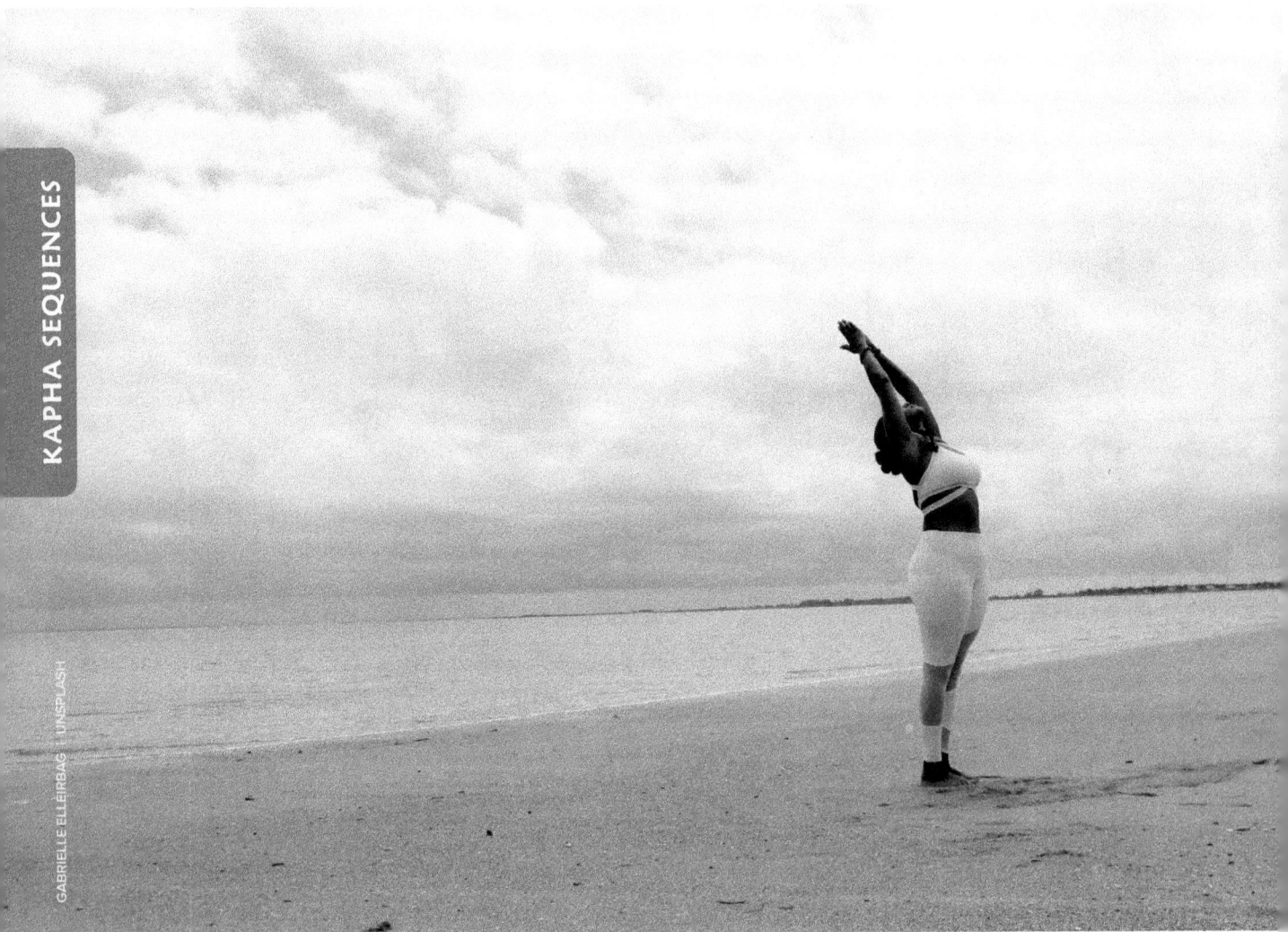

KAPHA SEQUENCES

Practice Sequences for Balancing Kapha

Home Site Practice for Kapha

Balancing kapha requires stimulating the lungs and diaphragm. Use the image of the kapha organs to refresh your memory about their location and shape.

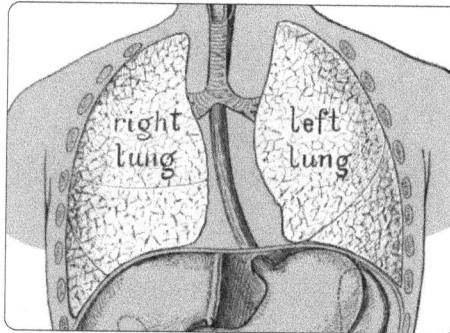

In doing the following kapha-balancing practices you can focus on the lungs and diaphragm themselves; or you can simply focus on opening the ribcage, enlivening the thoracic spine, and stimulating the area just below the bottom of the breastbone.

One focus is not inherently more effective, the one that you more easily connect to is the one to use.

continued

Home Site Practice, continued

🕐 35 - 40 minutes, whole practice

20-25 minutes — omit poses marked with *

10-12 minutes — do only poses marked with **

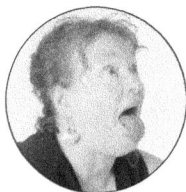

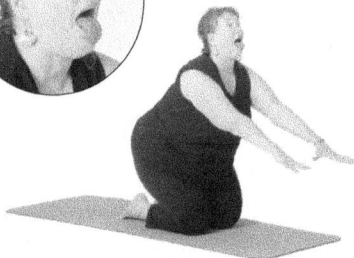

LION
Stretch through the mouth, tongue, lungs and stomach (option on stool). Repeat 3 times.

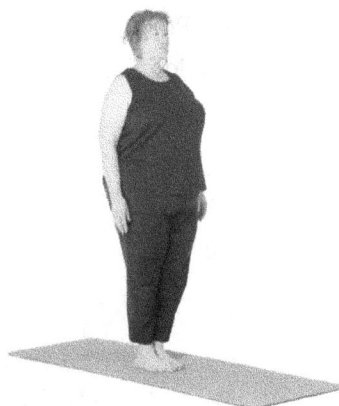

MOUNTAIN
Awaken upper spine, open the ribcage and lift the breastbone.

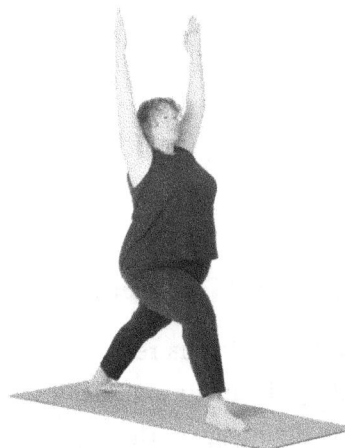

*HERO I (both sides)
Lift through the side ribs, opening the armpits and elongating the lungs.

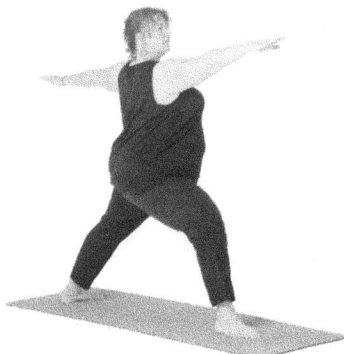

HERO 2 (both sides)
Widen the breastbone and ribs while expanding the lungs sideways.

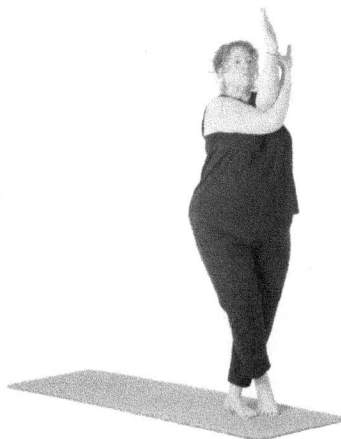

EAGLE ARMS
Widen the upper back and open the backs of the lungs.

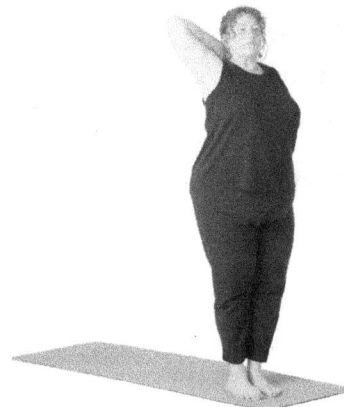

*COW'S FACE ARMS
Stretch and open the armpit ribs and elongate the sides of the lungs.

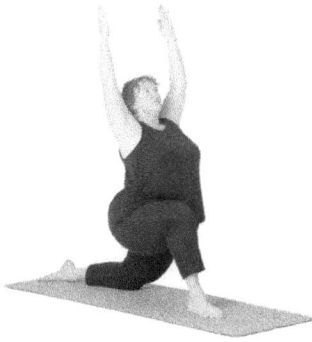

*MONKEY (both sides)
Stretch through the stomach, chest, upper back and arms.

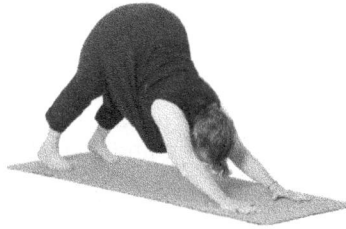

**DOWNWARD FACING DOG TO UPWARD FACING DOG
Elongate and vitalize the spine in both poses. Stretch through the stomach and lift the chest in the transition from Downward to Upward Dog. Repeat 4 times.

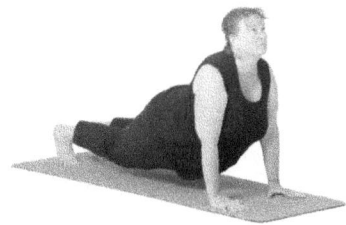

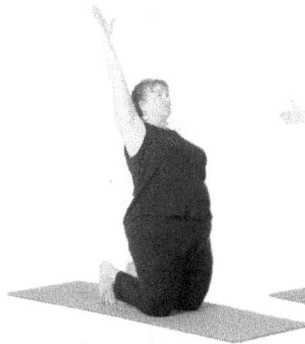

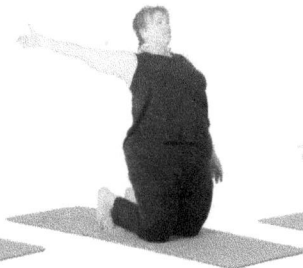

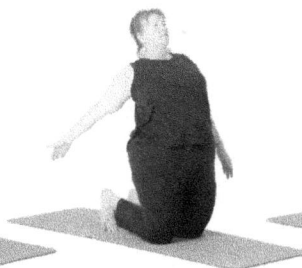

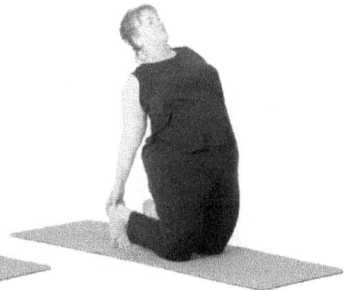

CAMEL One-sided with arm extension and spinal/rib rotation. Repeat on second side. Expand the chest, widen the collar bones, open the side ribs and spiral through the lungs.

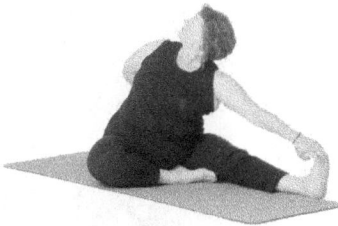

**SPINAL TWIST
Awaken a spiral through the ribs, upper spine, lungs and stomach.

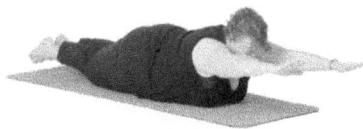

*DOWNWARD BOAT
Elongate the upper spine, stretch through the stomach and open space between the ribs using the reach of the arms and legs.

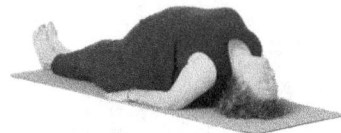

FISH
Spread the breastbone and blossom the fronts of the lungs.

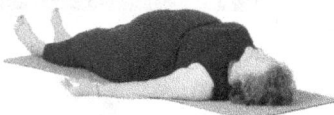

**SAVASANA

Heating Practice: Vinyasa

🕐 30 - 40 minutes

A vigorous vinyasa is heating and so is a good kapha–balancing option. You can use any sequence of asanas that allows for a relatively fast continuing flow of movement for 30 to 40 minutes. Sun salutations are good options; here is one variation to start with.

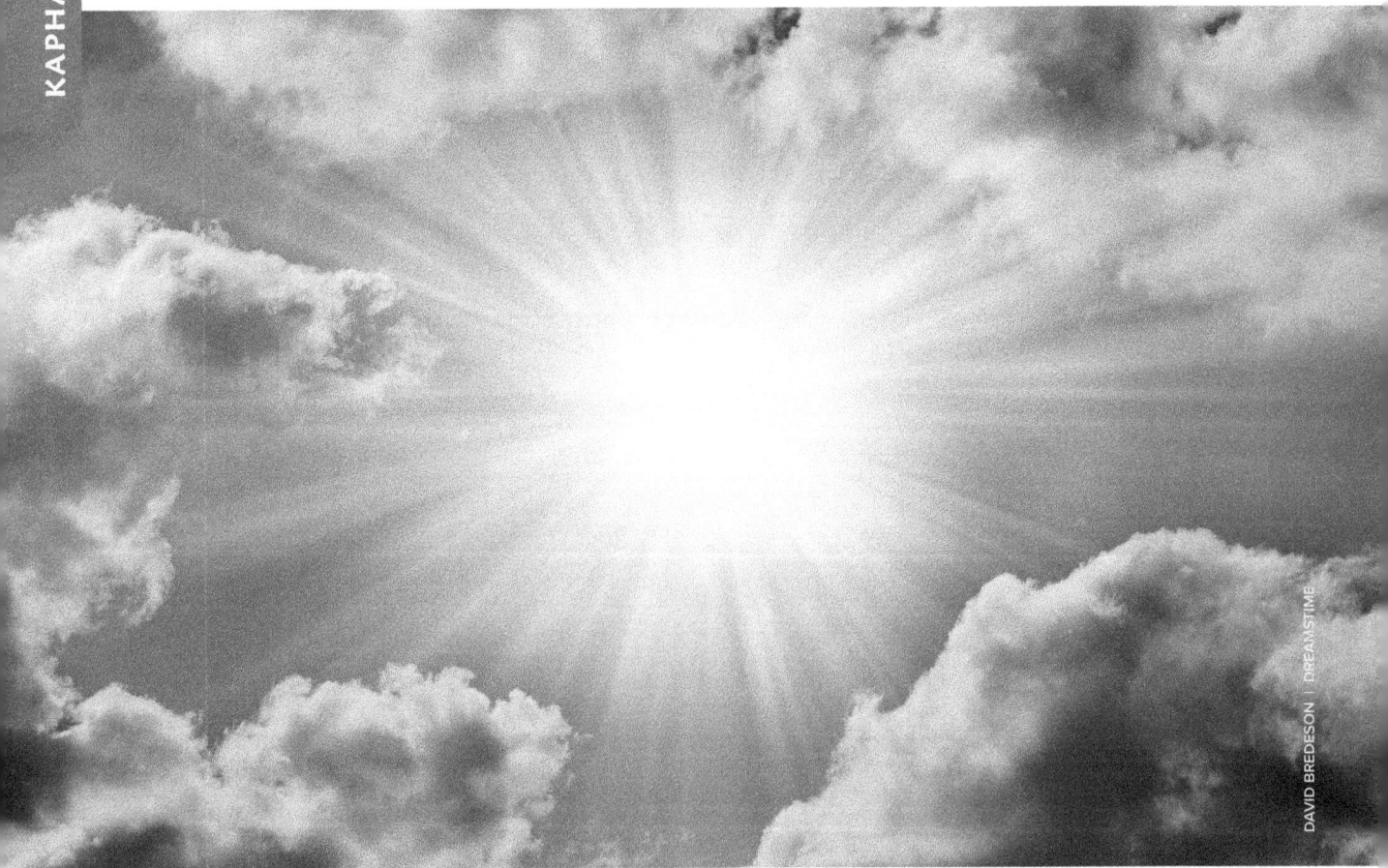

DAVID BREDESON | DREAMSTIME

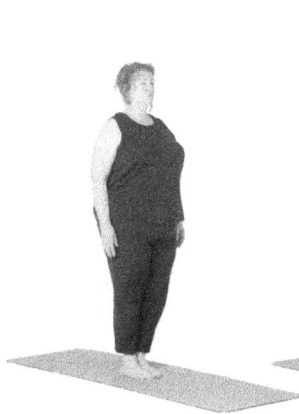

MOUNTAIN

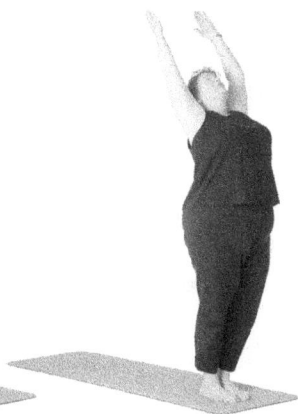

BACKBEND

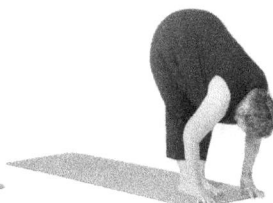

FORWARD BEND

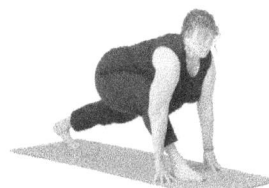

STRAIGHT LEG LUNGE

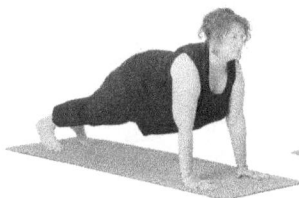

PLANK

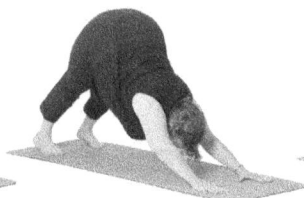

DOWNWARD FACING DOG

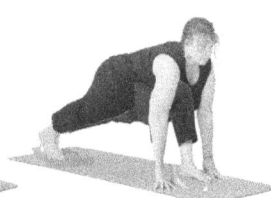

STRAIGHT LEG LUNGE

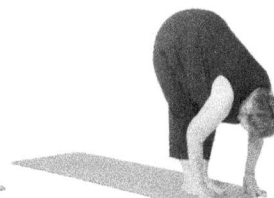

FORWARD BEND

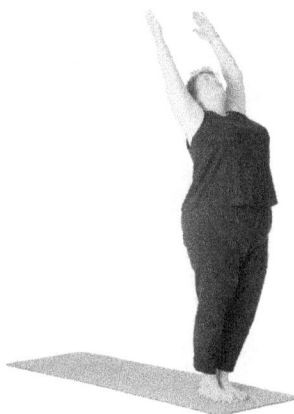

BACKBEND

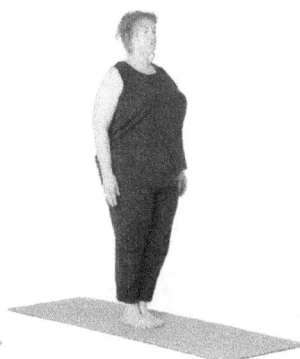

MOUNTAIN

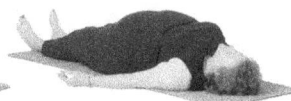

SAVASANA

Joints Practice: Create Space

🕐 30 - 35 minutes

20 - 25 minutes — to shorten practice, omit poses marked with *

Awakening the joints enlivens the whole body. In each of the following poses open space in the center of the joints. Maintain aware of your whole body as you cultivate space inside the joints.

Each of the poses has suggested joints on which to focus. Feel free to use fewer joints. As this process becomes more familiar you can include as many joints as you like.

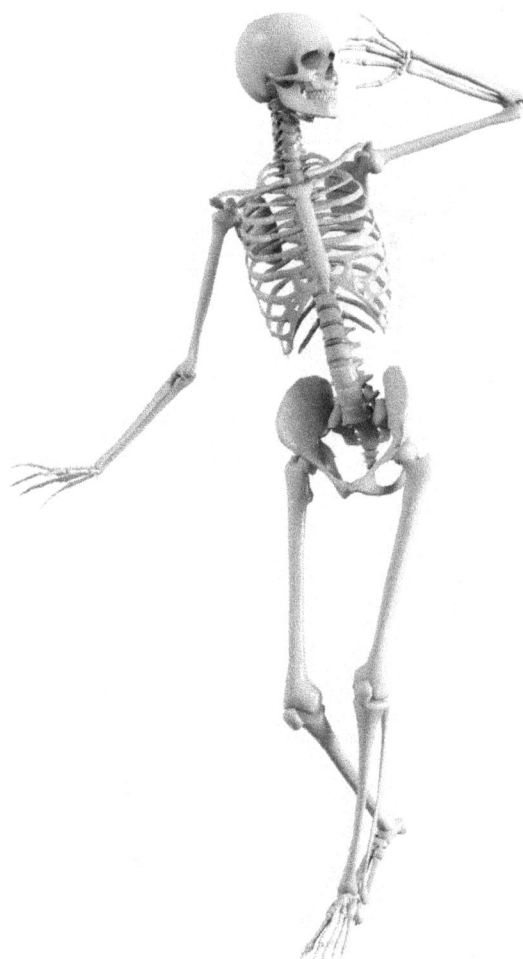

ANATERATE | PIXABAY

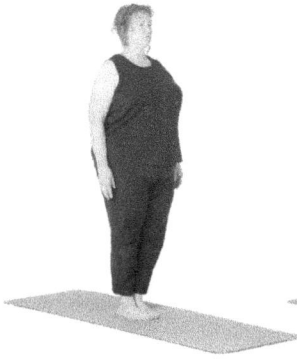

MOUNTAIN
Ankles and shoulders.

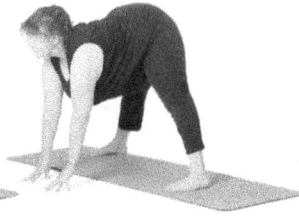

**STANDING
WIDE-LEGGED
FORWARD BEND**
Hips and shoulders.

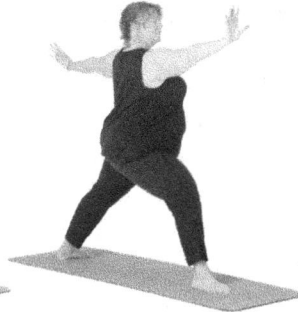

HERO II (both sides)
Front knee
and back ankle.

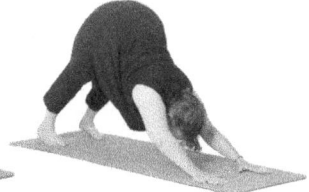

DOWNWARD DOG
Wrists and hip joints.

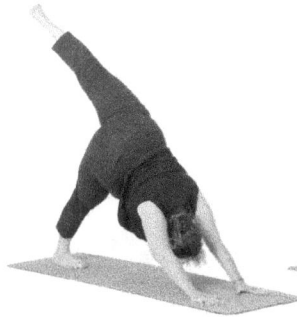

**DOWNWARD DOG
with leg extension**
Extended knee and
shoulders.

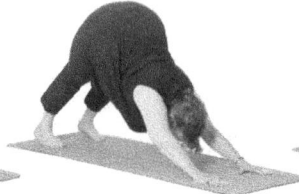

DOWNWARD DOG
Hip joints and
shoulder joints.

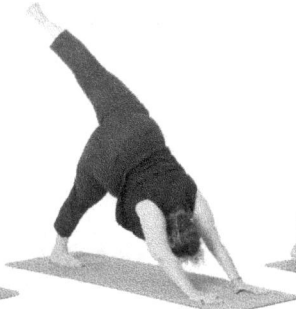

**DOWNWARD DOG
with leg extension**
(other leg) Extended leg
hips and shoulders.

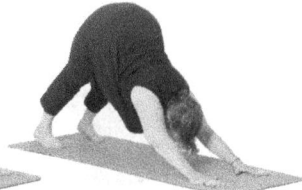

DOWNWARD DOG
Knees and elbows.

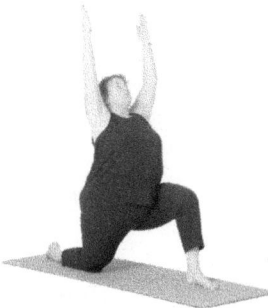

***MONKEY
(both sides)**
Back leg ankle and
front knee.

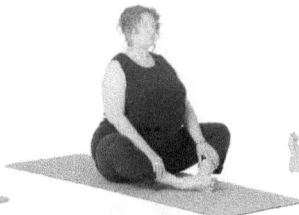

*BOUND ANGLE
Shoulder joints
and hip joints.

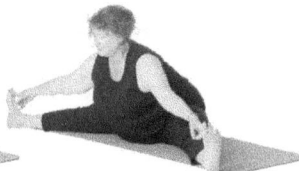

***SEATED
WIDE ANGLE
FORWARD BEND**
Shoulders and hips.

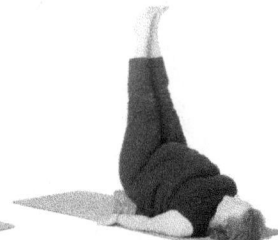

**HALF SHOULDER
STAND**
Ankles or knees
and shoulders.

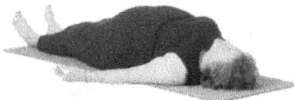

SAVASANA

Prana Practice: Engage Udana & Vyana

The upward movement of udana and the outward movement of vyana enliven kapha. This is a two-part practice and each part can be done separately or together.

🛈

Udana refresher on page 132.

Udana   🕐 10 minutes

In each of the following asanas, elongate the spine and lift the chest on the inhalation. Exhale as if the breath/udana is flowing from the area of the heart, through the neck and out through the crown of the head. Repeat each pose 3 times. Rest between each pose to allow the breath to settle.

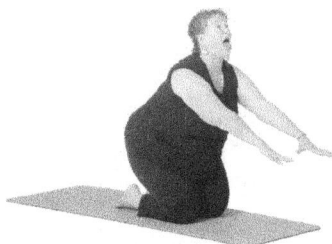

LION
Reach the tongue from deep in the throat and create a clear, full-throated, aspirated exhalation.

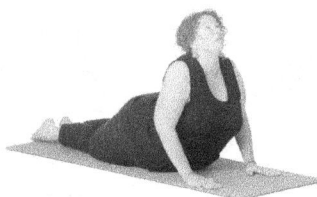

COBRA
Open the crown of the head as a channel for the exhalation.

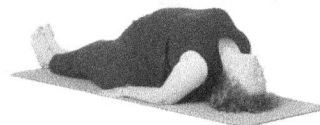

FISH
Relax the jaw, keep lips sealed and open the throat and nasal passages for the exhalation.

Rest briefly in Savasana before continuing.

Vyana ⏱ 10 minutes

Vyana refresher
on page 134.

In each of the following asanas, elongate the spine and lift the chest on
the inhalation. On the exhalation, let the breath flow as if from the heart
outward to and slightly beyond the surface of the body. If it is difficult
for you to hold your whole body in your awareness, start first by exhaling
outward from the heart though the ribcage, and then progressively
include more areas of the body.

Hold each pose as long as you feel at ease and can sustain your
awareness on the breath and vyana.

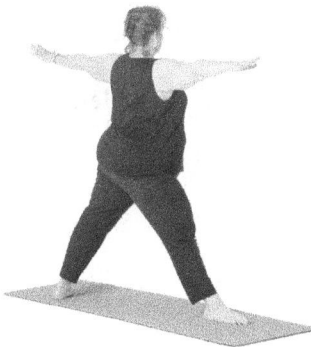

WIDE-LEGGED MOUNTAIN
with arm extensions

Elongate the spine and enliven the
crown of the head upward by imagining
it as a sunflower being attracted to the sun.

Hold the pose and turn your attention
to your breathing.

Lift the heart and exhale as if the breath is
flowing from the heart toward and slightly
beyond the surface of the body.

The inhalation is passive.

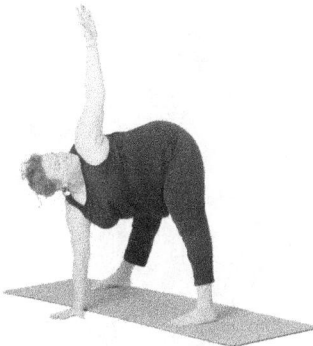

WIDE-LEG MOUNTAIN with
SPINAL TWIST (on both sides)

Repeat the process outlined above.

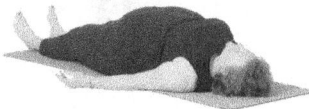

REST is Savasana.

Breath Practice: Stimulating Breath

🕐 12 - 15 minutes

Three Part Breath

Take a comfortable and stable seated position with your eyelids closed. Gently focus your eyes on the tip of your nose. Sit quietly until your body and breath are at ease.

Tune into the three-dimensional movement of the lungs as you breathe. Note that the top of the lungs are a bit above the collar bones.

◎ Inhale through the nose, filling the bottom of the lungs first, then fill the middle section of the lungs, and finally the top part of the lungs.

◎ In exhaling, first empty the lower lungs, next empty the middle of the lungs and finally the top of the lungs.

◎ Without strain, increase the size of the inhalation and exhalation with each breath. Encourage/allow a pause at the end of the inhalation and exhalation.

◎ Continue for 3 to 4 minutes.

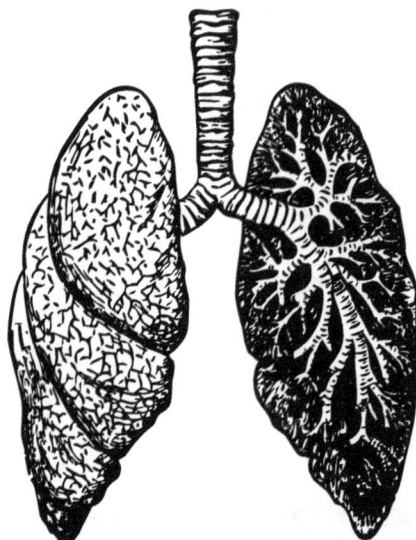

CLKER FREE VECTOR IMAGES | PIXABAY

Bastrika with Bridge Pose

◉ Take a Bridge pose that you can sustain with ease. Breathe with a strong bellows-like movement using equal-sized inhalations and exhalations (Bastrika*).

◉ Do 10 breaths and rest for 3 breaths.

◉ During the rest you can remain in Bridge pose or come out of it to rest.

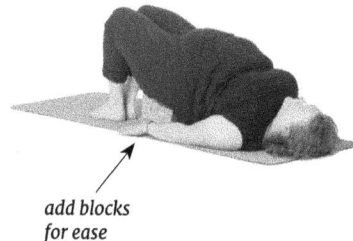

◉ Do 3 rounds.

add blocks for ease

Kapalabhati with One-Legged Bridge

◉ Take a One-Legged Bridge pose if you can sustain it with ease. If not use Bridge pose.

◉ Breathe with strong exhalations and passive inhalations (Kapalabhati breaths*).

◉ Hold the pose for 10 Kapalabhati breaths, and rest in Savasana for 3 - 5 breaths.

◉ Use the exhalations to enliven the arch of the spine and the extension of the leg.

◉ Do 3 rounds.

◉ Rest in Savasana.

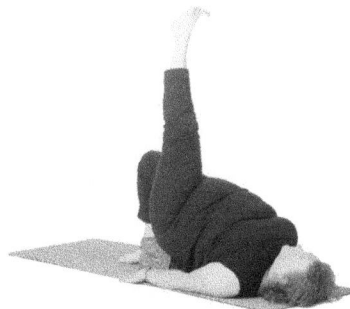

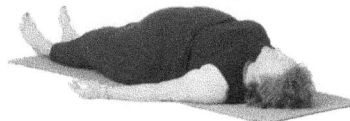

see Appendix, page 228

Meditation: Fire Imagery

🕐 10 - 20 minutes

Fire heats and balances kapha's cool nature.

◎ Take a comfortable seated position with your spine upright and alive but at ease. Have a lit candle placed a comfortable gazing distance in front of you.

◎ Awaken your body and breath with one cycle of Kapalabhati.*

◎ Gaze at the candle flame.

◎ Close your eyes and hold the image of the flame in your mind's eyes. Move the flame to your solar plexus — the 3rd chakra.

◎ Let each inhalation feed the flame so it grows hotter and stronger.

◎ Continue for 5 – 8 minutes.

◎ You can alternate between periods of rest and periods of feeding the flame.

◎ Rest quietly for a few moments before leaving the practice.

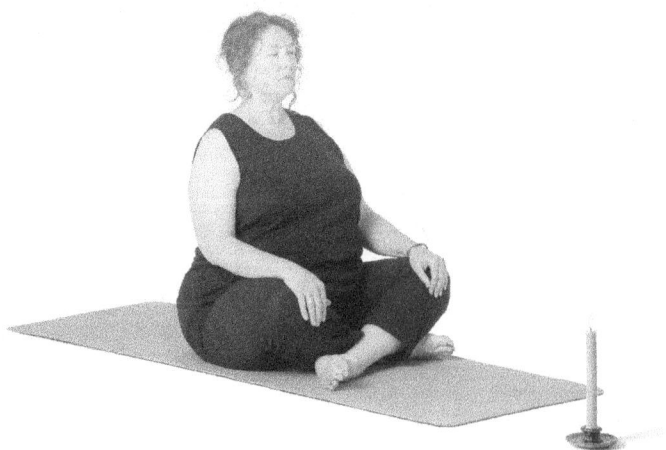

see Appendix, page 228

Acknowledgments

My deep gratitude to all of the teachers of yoga, Ayurveda and somatic awareness who influenced me in small and great ways. A special bow to Dr. Vasant Lad who presented Ayurveda to America.

A special note of appreciation for Karin Preus. The design of this book is central to making its content practical — and only by it being practical can it become meaningful. Karin's skill in design is obvious. That, coupled with her interest in expanding her own understanding of yoga and Ayurveda, brought a practitioner's aliveness and clarity to the design.

Karin applied her eye for detail to both the aesthetics and usability of this book. She rigorously tracked and cross-referenced material to make it easy for the reader to find related content. She contributed a third layer of editing by navigating stylistic accuracy together with the liberties we chose to take with the book in order to make it more user-friendly. All of this detail goes unnoticed because it recedes into the background, and allows the content to easily and clearly be available to the reader.

My warm appreciation to Cheryl Ekstrum, Mary Ann Bradley and Liz Liddiard Wozniak who open-heartedly agreed to be the models for respectively, vata, pitta and kapha.

The photographs of the models taken by Larry Marcus brought the dosha practices to life. The challenge of the photo shoots was made pleasant by his expertise, the charm of his loft studio and his quiet, unhurried willingness to take as many photos as necessary to get what we needed.

A special thanks to the accomplished people in the worlds of yoga, Ayurveda and somatic awareness whose words of support appear on the back cover.

I am grateful to Kevin Coughlin and Katie Charlet whose edits helped to polish this book. Additionally, Katie's grasp of the totality of the book reminded me not to get lost in detail, and Kevin's reliable presence created a welcome sense of support.

My appreciation to Gayle Burdick who spent a significant amount of time and energy editing the first iteration of this book which laid dormant for years and ultimately became the foundation for this book.

I am indebted to the photographers and models who generously offer their images without cost through Pexels.com and Unsplash.com. Their work made possible the visual beauty of this book and visual communication of the content.

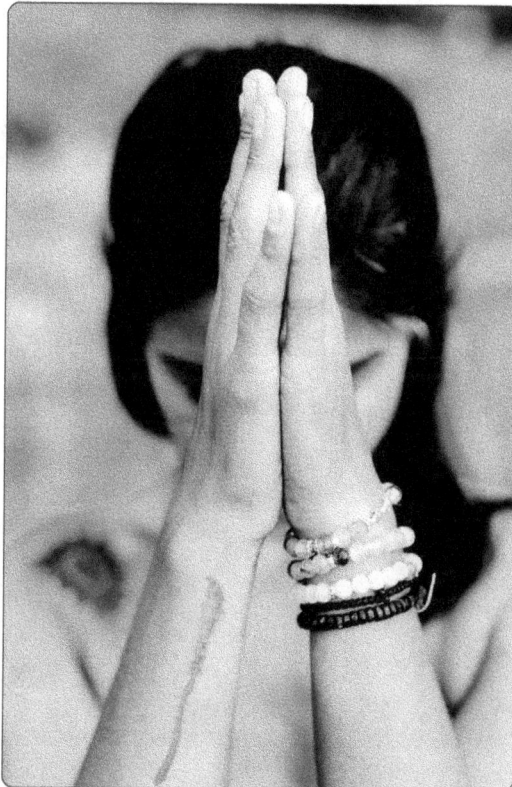

KIRILL PALII | UNSPLASH

Crown Chakra

Third Eye Chakra
Aum

Throat Chakra
Ham

Heart Chakra
Yam

Solar Plexus Chakra
Ram

Sacral Chakra
Vam

Root Chakra
Lam

Appendix

MORE on CHAKRAS

BIJ MANTRAS

Yoga and Ayurveda see the universe and everything within it as vibration. Mantras are a way of working with ourselves on the vibrational level. Mantras can be a syllable, a word or group of words. Seed mantras are single syllables. Seed mantras are also called bij mantras or seed/bij syllables.

Each of the seven major chakras has a seed mantra that can be used to create balance in the chakra, the element related to that chakra and all of the functions connected to that chakra.

You can repeat seed mantras out loud, sub-vocally or mentally.

Chanting seed mantras is most effective when done in a seated meditation position, but it is also useful to use them informally throughout the day to help us maintain a steady mind.

The "a" in all the seed sounds is pronounced as in "some."

MORE on BREATH PRACTICES

BASTRIKA and KAPALABHATI PRANAYAMAS

Bastrika and Kapalabhati are heating breath practices. They are normally done in a seated meditation posture but they can also be done together with asana. If you are not familiar with these practices it would be best to do them a few times in a seated position before working with them in asana. These breaths require a vigorous action of the torso and are contraindicated for high blood pressure, during menstruation or during pregnancy.

BASTRIKA (Bellows Breath)

Take a comfortable seated position with a grounded pelvis, released shoulders, relaxed, upright spine and hands resting on thighs. Let your eyes close and take a few moments to let the body and mind settle.

Breathe forcefully using an inhalation and exhalation that is of equal strength and duration. Maintain a stable spine and lifted chest throughout the practice, and engage the back and abdominal muscles in a harmonious, vigorous pumping action of the abdomen. Keep the lips sealed.

Do 3 rounds of 10 to 20 breaths. Rest between rounds letting your breath normalize. Respect your capacity.

KAPALABHATI (Skull Shining Breath)

Take a comfortable seated position with a grounded pelvis, released shoulders, relaxed, upright spine and hands resting on thighs. Let your eyes close and take a few moments to let the body and mind settle.

Breathe with strong, forceful exhalations and passive inhalations. Maintain a stable spine and lifted chest throughout the practice. Be aware of the alternating of the powerful abdominal action on the exhalation, and the release of the abdomen on the inhalation. Keep the lips sealed. Kapalabhati is considered a cleansing breath.

Do 3 rounds of 10 to 20 breaths. Rest between rounds letting your breath normalize. Respect your capacity.

SITALI and SITKARI

Sitali and Sitkari are cooling pranayamas. They are normally done in a seated meditation posture but they can also be done together with meditative asana. If you are not familiar with these practices it would be best to do them a few times in a seated position before working with them in asana.

SITALI

Take a comfortable seated position with a grounded pelvis, released shoulders, an easy upright spine with hands resting on thighs. Take a few moments to let the body and mind settle.

Curl the tongue into a lengthwise tube and thrust it out of the mouth. Inhale slowly and deeply across the surface of the curled tongue as if drinking through a straw. Sense the cooling sensation on the tongue and through the body. Do this for 1 or 2 minutes.

Rest quietly for a minute or so with a natural breath.

Repeat once or twice. Gradually increase the length of time.

SITKARI

Take a comfortable seated position with a grounded pelvis, released shoulders, relaxed, upright spine and hands resting on thighs. Take a few moments to let the body and mind settle.

Gently press your front upper and lower teeth together and stretch the corners of your lips straight to the side as much as you comfortably can, so you are exposing as many teeth as possible to the air. Inhale slowly through the spaces in the teeth and sense the coolness of the breath as it flows through the teeth, mouth and body.

Rest quietly for a minute or so with a natural breath.

Repeat once or twice. Gradually increase the length of time.

MORE ON DIGESTION

DIGESTIVE FIRE STRENGTHENERS

Agni Sara

A Guide to Agni Sara | Sandra Anderson

https://yogainternational.com/article/view/guide-to-agni-sara

Uddiyana Bandha

Uddiyana Bandha Step-by-Step | David Coulter

https://yogainternational.com/article/view/uddiyana-bandha-step-by-step

MORE ON HYPERMOBILITY

HYPERMOBILITY

Hypermobility is correlated with a number of seemingly unrelated problems among which are: anxiety, insomnia, autoimmune diseases, headaches, excess fatigue and digestive problems. It behooves people with any degree of hypermobility to learn more about associated problems.

Hypermobility ranges from a slight laxity in the joints, to extreme joint instability that is related to disease. For people who are on any part of the range of hypermobility it is important to be aware that focusing on increasing flexibility can actually stimulate problems. This awareness is crucial for teachers.

Here is the web address for getting a start on understanding the link between health problems and hypermobility.

https://www.nhsinform.scot/illnesses-and-conditions/muscle-bone-and-joints/conditions/joint-hypermobility#about-joint-hypermobility

Scott Anderson (scottandersonyoga.com) does research and consults clinically on hypermobility and health challenges. It was he who opened my eyes to the broader range of health problems correlated with hypermobility and suggested I expand my discussion on this topic. The scope of this book did not allow for more in-depth discussion so hopefully this short section will inspire people for whom it is relevant to further research this topic.

MORE ON SOMATIC AWARENESS

SOMATIC AWARENESS PIONEERS and the METHODS THEY CREATED

F.M. Alexander
The Alexander Technique
https://alexandertechnique.com/

Gerda Alexander
Eutony
https://eutony.co.uk/what–is–eutony/

Elsa Gindler
Somatic Awareness
https://www.returntooursenses.com/

Moshe Feldenkrais
The Feldenkrais Method
https://feldenkrais.com

MORE ON SOMATICS

From page 29:
www.somaticstudies.com/developmental-somatic-psychotherapy/definitions/

AYURVEDIC RESOURCES

From page 21:

*The Complete Book of
Ayurvedic Home Remedies*
Vasant Lad

Maharishi International University
Fairfield, Iowa
www.miu.edu

**National Ayurvedic Medicine
Association**
www.ayurvedanama.org

The Raj
Ayurvedic Health Center, Spa and Retreat
Fairfield, Iowa
www.theraj.com

Ayurvedic Institute
Albuquerque, New Mexico
www.ayurveda.com

MORE on the TWENTY QUALITIES of AYURVEDA

The TWENTY QUALITIES

The Qualities arise from the Elements, and so the Qualities are inherent in the doshas. Qualities are central in Ayurveda for both diagnosis and treatment.

What western medicine sees as a disease Ayurveda sees as a doshic disturbance. A doshic disturbance is made clearer and more specific through looking at imbalances in the Qualities. Qualities help to refine a diagnosis. Ayurvedic treatment uses the principle of balancing opposites for creating doshic balance, and in doing so it uses food, oils, sound, meditation, breathing practices, bodywork, asana and special preparations based on their qualities.

A Western mind may have difficulty grasping the healing potential of something so seemingly ordinary as twenty qualities. Once we delve more deeply into this perspective, however, we find a profound intelligence. The richness, complexity and possibility in this view begin to unfold.

In this book I briefly describe some of the qualities because they are essential in understanding the Elements and the Doshas. The scope of this book does not allow for describing all the qualities or working with them in any depth so, following is a bit more detail for those who are interested.

The TWENTY QUALITIES (Gunas)

There are twenty qualities and they function as pairs of opposites that are used to balance each other. Each pair can also be looked at as a continuum.

Twenty Gunas as Opposites		Ten Continua
Heavy	Light	Weight
Dense	Liquid	Fluid content
Slow	Sharp	Capacity to penetrate
Soft	Hard	Capacity to yield or resist
Cold	Hot	Temperature
Static	Mobile	Motion and mobility
Oily	Dry	Lubrication
Subtle	Gross	Permeability
Smooth	Rough	Texture
Cloudy	Clear	Perception

continued

QUALITIES and the DOSHAS

Below are sketched out a few possibilities of where and how the qualities can express in the doshas. They can be a start for looking at ourselves through the lens of qualitative awareness, and to cultivate qualitative thinking.

VATA QUALITIES and POSSIBLE EXPRESSIONS

Cold — body temperature, easily chilled, emotions

Dry — skin, hair, sense of humor, muscles, bones

Light — weight, emotions, attitude

Rough — skin, nails, awkward movements

Subtle — vagueness, capacity to grasp subtlety in thoughts and emotions

Mobile/Quick — excess mobility in joints, moving quickly, creative, dispersed thinking,

Clear — clarity of thoughts and emotions, psychic ability

PITTA QUALITIES and POSSIBLE EXPRESSIONS

Hot — body, emotions, passion, temper

Sharp/Penetrating — thoughts, tongued (as in speech), perceptive mind

Light — brightness of mind and personality

Oily — skin, hair

Spreading — networking, powerful communicating

Liquid — regulates heat, spreads heat, cohesive

KAPHA QUALITIES and POSSIBLE EXPRESSIONS

Heavy — stability, lethargy

Dense — difficult to penetrate, strength

Slow — not rushing, not being able to get moving, patience

Cold — solidifying, slows digestion

Soft — emotions, heart

Oily — soft skin, lubrication of joints

Smooth — easing transitions, lubricates

Cloudy — emotional and mental lack of clarity

Static — unable to get moving, good grounding

Hard — insensitivity, rigidity, strength

Gross — resistant, thickness

Some of the qualities are in just one dosha, and some are in two doshas. The influence of a quality that is present in two doshas will vary depending on the presence or absence of other qualities.

A yoga practice organized around qualities is organic and process-oriented, rather than linear and goal-oriented. The key is allowing time for exploring a quality, and being receptive to how it unfolds in your body/mind and practice.

EXPLORING the TWENTY QUALITIES

Here are a few ways to explore yourself through the lens of the Qualities.

Noticing Your Internal Qualities

- Can you describe a few of your familiar emotional states using the qualities?
- What qualities arise in you after an experience that nourishes you?
- What qualities arise in you after participating in an activity that you find depleting?

Noticing External Qualities

- What qualities do you like in food? What qualities do you dislike?
- What qualities are you attracted to in people?
- Are there particular qualities that attract you to social situations, e.g., mobile (dancing, tennis) or subtle (philosophical conversation)?

Bringing Qualities into Your Practice Space

Choose an image or object that expresses qualities you would like to cultivate and place it in your practice space. You can meditate on the image and the qualities, or you can allow them to be a felt-sense that you periodically bring into focus.

Faye Berton

Faye has been teaching yoga and working with The Feldenkrais Method® since 1988. She has the highest certification from Yoga Alliance and is a FGNA Feldenkrais practitioner. She is a certified Ayurvedic Lifestyles Consultant through the Ayurvedic Institute, was published in *Light on Ayurveda*, and is currently on the board of the Minnesota Ayurveda Association.

Her studies in yoga philosophy were primarily through The Himalayan Tradition as taught by Swami Nijananda Bharati and Swami Veda Bharati. Her training in asana is extensive and varied. Some of the world's masters of somatic disciplines with whom she has trained include Marjorie Barstow, Emilie Conrad, Charlotte Selver, Else Middendorf and Ruthy Alon.

After establishing the Laurel Yoga Studio in St. Paul, Minnesota, she moved to Mexico and opened the Casa Lalita Retreat Center. For many years she taught between Mexico, USA and Canada. After 23 years of teaching asana, she developed the Fluid Strength Yoga Practice. She now lives in St. Paul, where she teaches Fluid Strength, does private sessions in The Feldenkrais Method, and develops health and wellness workshops.

She also authored a book on the practice she developed, *The Fluid Strength Yoga Practice: Vitalizing the Body and Resting the Mind*.

www.faye-berton.com

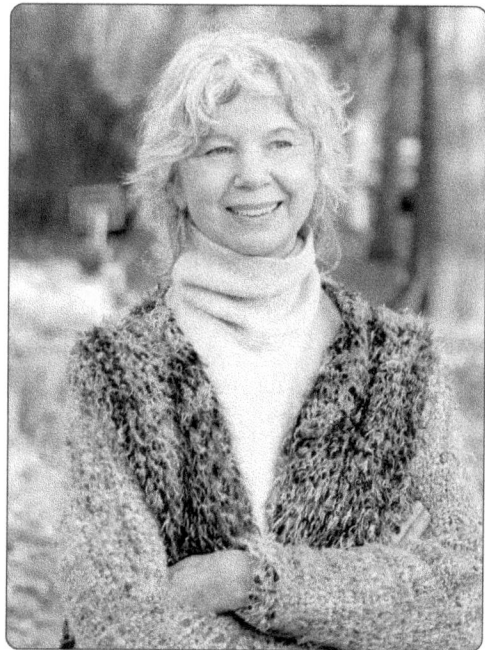

LARRY MARCUS